KT-430-863

Psychological Disorders in Obstetrics and Gynaecology for the MRCOG and Beyond

Published titles in this series

Antenatal Disorders for the MRCOG and Beyond *by Andrew Thomson and Ian Greer*

Fetal Medicine for the MRCOG and Beyond *by Alan Cameron, Lena Macara, Janet Brennand and Peter Milton*

Gynaecological and Obstetric Pathology for the MRCOG *by Harold Fox and C. Hilary Buckley, with a chapter on Cervical Cytology by Dulcie V. Coleman*

Gynaecological Oncology for the MRCOG and Beyond *edited by David Luesley and Nigel Acheson*

Gynaecological Urology for the MRCOG and Beyond *by Simon Jackson, Meghana Pandit and Alexandra Blackwell*

Haemorrhage and Thrombosis for the MRCOG and Beyond *edited by Anne Harper*

Intrapartum Care for the MRCOG and Beyond *by Thomas F. Baskett and Sabaratnam Arulkumaran, with a chapter on Neonatal Resuscitation by John McIntyre and a chapter on Perinatal Loss by Carolyn Basak*

Management of Infertility for the MRCOG and Beyond *by Allan A. Templeton et al.*

Menopause for the MRCOG and Beyond *by Margaret Rees*

Medical Genetics for the MRCOG and Beyond *by Michael Connor*

Menstrual Problems for the MRCOG *by Mary Ann Lumsden, Jane Norman and Hilary Critchley*

Neonatology for the MRCOG *by Peter Dear and Simon Newell*

Reproductive Endocrinology for the MRCOG and Beyond *edited by Adam Balen*

The MRCOG: A Guide to the Examination *by Ian Johnson et al.*

Forthcoming titles in the series

Early Pregnancy Issues

Molecular Medicine

Psychological Disorders in Obstetrics and Gynaecology for the MRCOG and Beyond

Khaled MK Ismail MD MRCOG
Senior Lecturer/Consultant in Obstetrics and Gynaecology, Academic Unit of
Obstetrics and Gynaecology, Keele University Medical School, University
Hospital of North Staffordshire, Stoke-on-Trent ST4 6QG, UK

Ilana Crome MD FRCPsych
Professor of Addiction Psychiatry, Academic Psychiatry Unit, Keele University
Medical School, Harplands Hospital, Stoke-on-Trent ST4 6TH, UK

PM Shaughn O'Brien MD FRCOG
Professor of Obstetrics and Gynaecology, Academic Unit of Obstetrics and
Gynaecology, Keele University Medical School, University Hospital of North
Staffordshire, Stoke-on-Trent ST4 6QG, UK

Series Editor: Jennifer Higham FRCOG

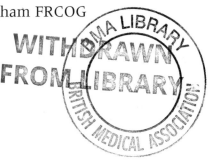

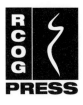

Published by the **RCOG Press** at the Royal College of Obstetricians and
Gynaecologists, 27 Sussex Place, Regent's Park, London NW1 4RG

www.rcog.org.uk

Registered charity no. 213280

First published 2006

ISBN 1-904752-09-8

RCOG Editor: Jane Moody
Design/typesetting by Karl Harrington, FiSH Books, London
Index by Liza Furnival, Medical Indexing Ltd

Printed by Latimer Trend & Co. Ltd, Estover Road, Plymouth PL6 7PL, UK

Cover illustration: © 2006 JupiterImages corporation

Acknowledgements
The authors would like to thank Miss Corrina Knight, Research Secretary at the
Academic Psychiatry Unit, Keele University Medical School, for her administrative and
secretarial support.

Contents

Abbreviations

ACTH	adrenocorticotrophic hormone
BMI	body mass index
CNS	central nervous system
CRH	corticotrophin-releasing hormone
CTG	cardiotocogram
DSM-IV	*Diagnostic and Statistical Manual of Mental Health* 4th edition
ECG	electrocardiogram
EPDS	Edinburgh Postnatal Depression Scale
ESR	erythrocyte sedimentation rate
FSH	follicle-stimulating hormone
GABA	gamma amino butyric acid
GABA-A	gamma amino butyric acid type A
GnRH	gonadotrophin-releasing hormone
HFEA	Human Fertilisation and Embryology Authority
HPA	hypothalamic-pituitary-adrenal system
HRT	hormone replacement therapy
ICD-10	*International Classification of Diseases*, 10th edition
IQ	intelligence quotient
LH	luteinising hormone
LLPDD	late luteal phase dysphoric disorder
MAO	monoamine oxidase
MAOIs	monoamine oxidase inhibitors

NaSSA	noradrenergic and specific serotonergic antidepressant
NICE	National Institute for Clinical Excellence
PMDD	premenstrual dysphoric disorder
PMS	premenstrual syndrome
PSST	premenstrual symptoms screening tool
RCTs	randomised controlled trials
SAD	seasonal affective disorder
SNRI	serotonin-noradrenaline reuptake inhibitor
SSRI	selective serotonin reuptake inhibitor
TACE	tolerance, annoyed, cut down, eye opener
TRH	thyrotrophin-releasing hormone
TSH	thyroid-stimulating hormone

Introduction

Psychological disorders remain among the most highly stigmatised conditions in medical practice. Women may suffer, knowingly or unknowingly. Perhaps this is the major reason why the 2000–2002 report of the Confidential Enquiries into Maternal Deaths uncovered the startling finding that, when all deaths up to 1 year after delivery were taken into account, psychiatric illness was not only the leading indirect cause of death but also the leading cause of maternal deaths overall.[1]

This outcome can be the result of lack of access to appropriate services, inadequate assessment, recognition and diagnosis, ineffective treatment, inconsistent review and monitoring of the interventions that have been implemented, and poor coordination between services.

This book attempts to redress the balance. It covers the psychological conditions associated with the many phases of the woman's life span: menarche, menstrual disorders, pregnancy and menopause. In parallel, but linked with cross-referencing, it aims to outline the main psychological comorbid symptoms or syndromes with which women may present.

The highlight is on description of the nature and extent of the parti cular condition, detection or diagnosis, the pharmacological and psychosocial interventions available and the importance of referral to and co-working with multidisciplinary teams. Substance misuse, mood disorders, severe mental illness, eating disorders, personality problems, suicide and deliberate self-harm are considered.

We highlight the growing evidence base for treatment for psychiatric disorder. It is important to underline the rapid scientific advances in mental health in general and in relation to obstetrics and gynaecology, through an understanding of the neurosciences, linked to psychosocial influences, and to the higher priority given to mental health in the national policy agenda.

For all these reasons we hope to stress how you can intervene effectively by pointing to how you can recognise and treat directly or refer those women whom you suspect have a primary or secondary associated mental disorder.

DEFINITIONS

Psychiatry	A branch of medicine concerned with the study and treatment of mental illness and behavioural disturbance.
Psychiatrist	A medical practitioner specialising in the diagnosis and treatment of mental illness.
Psychology	The scientific study of the human mind and its functions.
	The mental characteristics or attitude of a person.
	Mental factors governing a situation or activity.
Psychotherapy	The treatment of mental disorder by psychological rather than medical means.
Psychosocial	The inter-relationship of social factors and individual thought and behaviour.

Reference

1. Lewis G, editor. *Why Mothers Die 2000–2002. The Sixth Report of the Confidential Enquiries into Maternal Deaths in the United Kingdom.* London: RCOG Press; 2004.

1 Diagnosis and management of psychological problems

Introduction

This chapter outlines the common types of psychological problems, the principles of assessment, pharmacological modalities, psychological interventions and particular problems of special groups of people. Later chapters outline where endocrine and even surgical interventions, in rare situations, may be relevant.

The largest cause of maternal deaths overall is psychiatric illness and, of the 391 women whose deaths were reported to the Confidential Enquiries into Maternal Deaths in the United Kingdom in 2000–2002, 8% were substance misusers (Figure 1.1).[1]

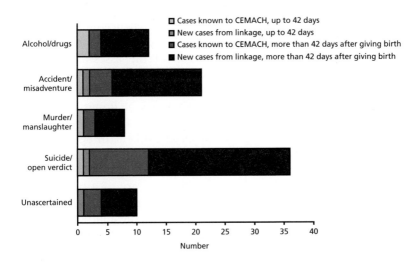

Figure 1.1 Maternal deaths from psychiatric, accidental, violent of unascertained causes; England and Wales 2000–02; reproduced with permission from CEMACH[1]

Health professionals must have a sound knowledge of the adverse consequences of mental illness in order to detect, treat and provide care. Psychological symptoms and psychological syndromes that often go unnoticed can have serious implications for the woman, her family and health practitioners. It is the role of the obstetrician and gynaecologist to be aware of the symptoms of common syndromes, always to consider the possibility of coexisting psychological problems and to make a diagnosis where they are reasonably confident or request support when necessary. In summary, the obstetrician and gynaecologist has a duty to have a high index of suspicion with regard to psychological problems. Similarly, it is important for psychiatrists and other healthcare professionals to be aware of the physiological and psychological processes specifically related to obstetrics and gynaecology.

Psychological problems may pre-date, be associated with or be precipitated by obstetric or gynaecological problems. Women may actually present with a range of different symptoms. However, they may also find it difficult to admit to and access help and support for specific psychological problems, even if they or their families do recognise their problems.

General principles of assessment

The ability to carry out an assessment in an empathic, non-judgemental manner is essential for the success of any treatment. Further management should be based on the clinician's balanced interpretation of consistency between the systematic history, clinical condition and results of investigations. Communication of the assessment to the woman, her family and relevant professionals (with consent) is part of the process. It is important to recognise that there may be a psychological component to the presentation, so it may be important to refer to other medical specialists, such as psychiatrists and their teams, other professions, such as psychologists and social workers, or agencies such as social services.

A high index of suspicion is vital. First and foremost, it is crucial to determine if the woman is already under the care of a physician or psychiatrist or receiving pharmacological treatment or psychological interventions. If so, contact should be made with the appropriate teams with the woman's agreement. Furthermore, unexplained physical symptoms should alert the obstetrician to the possibility of psychological difficulties and the need to review and monitor perhaps unnecessary investigations. The past psychiatric history of the woman is also relevant. The use of the Mental Health Act should be cautiously probed if you think this might have been an issue at any time. Stressors such as bereavement, unemployment, promotion, physical and sexual abuse, bullying, harassment, recent marriage, separation or divorce may predispose people to the development of psychological and physical problems.

It is important to try to determine aspects of the family background or social circumstances that may be pertinent: past or current psychiatric illness, including treatment (particularly current drug treatment), admission, response to treatment in a close relative (parents, siblings, children, grandparents, aunts or uncles).

The woman must be treated with respect and courtesy. Ensure that she recognises that you are there to support improvement in her health function. During the consultation give her and her relatives time, so that they can express themselves in their way, listen with understanding, be reassuring, make eye contact and use their names. Try not to use technical language, explain what you mean if you do so, and couch it in a way that does not appear patronising. If the woman is irate, taxing, seductive or inquisitive, try not to take it personally and respond politely, with understanding. At the same time, be firm and clear with regard to the nature of the relationship, which is professional.

If appropriate, an overall assessment of the general level of functioning in educational and occupational domains, relationships with parents, her peers, her partner, children, colleagues and professionals, should be sought.

Would you describe this person's situation as stable, chaotic, deteriorating, improving, a cause for concern or a contributory factor to their mental or physical state? Is the woman well supported by a network of family, friends and professionals? Is the woman living in suitable accommodation? Is the woman homeless? Is the woman a lone parent, a widow or living alone? Is there concern, anxiety, evidence or suspicion of domestic violence, substance misuse, legal difficulties or criminal activities?

Investigations should be appropriately targeted. Unless these are clearly necessary to clarify a diagnosis, one should be aware there is always the possibility that the woman is being over-investigated.

Diagnostic categories

PSYCHOSIS

Schizophrenia is the most common psychotic disorder. It is characterised by abnormal perceptions, beliefs, thought processing and volition. There are acute and chronic forms. In the acute type, auditory and bodily (somatic) hallucinations, delusions, thought insertion and withdrawal, as well as passivity experiences can occur. In the chronic form, negative symptoms: apathy, blunted affect, social withdrawal, self-neglect and poverty of thought and speech, are manifest.

AFFECTIVE SYMPTOMS

There are two kinds of mood disorder: mania and depression.

Mania

This state can develop rapidly; that is, over days, and results in elation, grandiosity, overactivity, disinhibition and exhaustion as well as lability of mood. Psychotic symptoms accompany mania.

Depression

Depression is characterised by physical and psychological symptoms. The psychological problems include low mood, lability of mood, irritability, self-blame and guilt, feelings of hopelessness and helplessness and loss of interest. The physical difficulties include fatigue, lack of energy, poor sleep, poor appetite, weight loss, agitation or retardation, loss of libido and dehydration. In addition, women may suffer from inability to concentrate and complain of memory loss.

Sometimes depression is associated with psychotic symptoms such as delusions or hallucinations. The most serious risk is that of suicide.

SUICIDE AND DELIBERATE SELF-HARM

Deliberate self-harm refers to harm that does not result in death but is a way of coping with distressing feelings. This may occur in a state of crisis, stress or worsening mental state and psychiatric symptoms. Women attempt suicide more often than men but men complete suicide more often than women (Figure 1.2). Suicide rates for men, which were rising through the 1970s and 1980s, have decreased steadily since 1998. The rate for 2003, 18.1 deaths/100 000 population, was the lowest since 1978. Suicide rates for women, which fell steadily in the 1980s and early 1990s, have decreased only slightly since the mid-1990s. The rate for women remained around 5.8 deaths/100 000 population in each of the years 2001 to 2003.

Single, divorced or widowed people are more likely to attempt suicide than those who are married. Stressful life events such as job loss, bereavement and financial difficulties are associated with suicide. Caring for a child is protective. Unsuccessful attempts in the past make it more likely that a future attempt will be successful. Substance misuse

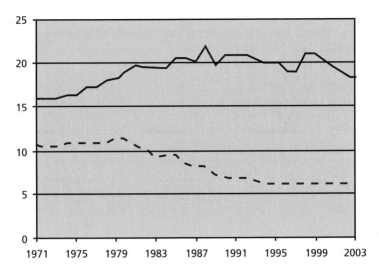

Figure 1.2 Suicide rates per 1000 population for men and women in the UK (Source: Office for National Statistics); — = men; ---- = women

is a powerful predictor of deliberate self-harm and suicide. An overdose may not be accidental and the assessment should always explore underlying suicidal intent or maladaptive coping responses.

Depression, bipolar disorder, personality disorder and psychotic illness may be associated with deliberate self-harm and with eventual suicide.

ANXIETY

Anxiety presents as recurrent, inappropriate, unrealistic, intrusive and irrational fear. There are several sorts of anxiety disorder; that is, panic, agoraphobia, social phobia, generalised anxiety disorder, obsessive-compulsive disorder and post-traumatic stress disorder.

POST-TRAUMATIC STRESS DISORDER

Women may have experienced such severe levels of abuse – physical, sexual or psychological – or other stressful experiences, that they develop a diagnosable condition.

Importantly for the purpose of this book, people may present with specific fears relating to their health; that is, unexplained somatic complaints or hypochondriacal disorder. Of course, anxiety itself may be accompanied by many somatic symptoms, which may mimic physical disorders. These include sweating, dry mouth, palpitations, tremor, hyperventilation, headache, backache, flushing, nausea, diarrhoea, urinary frequency and muscular tension.

PERSONALITY DISORDERS

Personality disorders are primary disorders. The features are recognisable by adolescence and persist. They are defined as maladaptive patterns of behaviour that cause distress and difficulties in social functioning which impact on the individual and others. There are several kinds of personality disorder; for example, paranoid, schizoid, dissocial, emotionally unstable, histrionic, obsessional, anxious and dependent.

ACUTE ORGANIC BRAIN REACTION (DELIRIUM OR CONFUSIONAL STATE)

This is characterised by:

- impaired consciousness
- poor attention; that is, disorientation for time, place or person
- illusions, hallucinations, delusions
- overactivity, restlessness, agitation
- emotional lability
- drowsiness and insomnia
- perplexity
- suspiciousness.

DIETING DISORDERS

Dieting disorders include anorexia nervosa and bulimia nervosa. Both are associated with serious psychiatric and physical disturbances. In both, individuals adopt restricted eating patterns and excessive dieting disorders. Sufferers over-evaluate their shape and weight as a marker of self-worth.

In anorexia nervosa there is an unduly low body weight, while in bulimia nervosa there is recurrent bingeing, vomiting and laxative use.

Anorexia nervosa may result in amenorrhoea, dry skin, fine downy hair, fatigue, abdominal discomfort, headaches, stunted growth, hypothermia, hypotension, brachycardia and arrhythmias, hyperactivity, brittle bones and osteoporosis. Dental decay, polyuria, paresthesia, stress fractures and swollen salivary glands occur because of the behavioural problems.

In bulimia, a range of problems result: amenorrhoea, dental decay, irritable bowel, nausea, fatigue, headaches, insomnia, hair loss, callused knuckles, urinary tract infections, bruising and swollen hands, feet and salivary glands.

As will be apparent, these symptoms overlap with those of depression, personality disorders, obsessional symptoms, and gastrointestinal disorders.

General principles of treatment

PSYCHIATRIC DISORDERS AND DRUG TREATMENT

'Older' antipsychotics

Antipsychotic medication (neuroleptics or major tranquillisers) is the main form of medication. These drugs reduce relapse, the most common reason for which is non-compliance. 'Classical' antipsychotics, such as chlorpromazine, thioridazine, sulpiride, act on 'positive' symptoms. There are depot injections available. They are used for schizophrenia, mania and organic brain syndromes.

Atypical antipsychotics

These act on both the 'positive' acute symptoms and 'negative' symptoms. Examples of these drugs are clozapine, risperidone, olanzapine, quetiapine and amisulpiride. These drugs do not have the anticholinergic and extrapyramidal adverse effects of the older drugs. However, some, such as weight gain, seizures, sedation, dizziness and agranulocytosis, are common to both.

Antidepressant medication

There is a large range of antidepressant medication available. These include:

- tricyclic, e.g. amitriptyline, clomipramine, dosulepin (dothiepin), doxepin, imipramine, lofepramine, nortriptyline, trimipramine

- tetracyclic, e.g. mianserin, maprotiline, amoxapine

- selective serotonin reuptake inhibitors (SSRIs), e.g. citalopram, sertraline, fluoxetine, fluvoxamine, paroxetine

- monoamine oxidase inhibitors (MAOIs), e.g. isocarboxazid, phenelzine, tranylcypromine, moclobemide

- serotonin-noradrenaline reuptake inhibitors (SNRIs), e.g. venlafaxine

- post-synaptic serotonin receptor blockers and reuptake inhibitors, e.g. trazodone

- noradrenergic/specific serotonergic antidepressants (NaSSA), e.g. mirtazapine.

These are variously used for depression, panic disorder, obsessive–compulsive disorder and bulimia nervosa.

Lithium, sodium valproate and carbamazepine are also used for the prophylaxis and treatment of mania and depression, alone or in combination.

Benzodiazepines

Benzodiazepines are used as hypnotics, sedatives or anxiolytics. There are many types, with different half-lives. It is important to recognise that they can produce a withdrawal syndrome, i.e. dependence, even if low doses have been prescribed (or misused). If taken in combination with other drugs and alcohol, overdose can result. There are alternatives, such as buspirone, zolpidem and zopiclone, which can be used and do not appear to lead to dependence.

DRUG USE IN PREGNANCY AND BREASTFEEDING

These are covered in Chapter 6.

PSYCHOLOGICAL INTERVENTIONS

A wide range of effective interventions is available. These interventions may be brief or intensive and delivered in community, primary care, outpatient or inpatient settings, by specialist psychiatrists and mental health teams, and by general practitioners and their teams. They may be for an individual, in a group setting or for a family (Box 1.1).

Brief, minimal and short-term interventions, including 'counselling' and 'motivational interviewing' have become popular and the latter is developing a growing evidence base.

BOX 1.1 COMMONLY USED PSYCHOLOGICAL
INTERVENTIONS:

• Non-directive counselling
• Cognitive behavioural approach
• Social network behaviour therapy
• Family therapy
• Motivational interviewing

Psychological approaches

BOX 1.2. IMPORTANT COMMON OBJECTIVES OF
PSYCHOLOGICAL TREATMENTS

Problem solving	Developing competence in dealing with a specific problem
Acquisition of social skills	Mastery of social and interpersonal skills by assertiveness or anger control
Cognitive change	Modification of irrational beliefs and maladaptive patterns of thought
Behaviour change	Modification of maladaptive behaviour
Systemic change	Introducing change into family systems

INFORMATION-BASED METHODS

It should be borne in mind that there is considerable evidence from other health and social care fields that health education and the provision of information, in itself, may be of help, especially in less complex situations. Information needs to be accurate and up to date and should provide positive advice.

COUNSELLING

'Counselling' is a widely used term, which can be imprecise and which can embody different theoretical models, such as psychodynamic, cognitive or behavioural. In practice, however, counselling may have one or more objectives: problem solving, acquisition of social skills, cognitive change, behavioural or systemic change. The term may be used to describe therapies that are supportive, directive or motivational, for individuals, groups or families. The term may encompass assessment, engagement and support, together with the development of therapeutic relationships. Box 1.2 shows important common objectives.

NONDIRECTIVE COUNSELLING

In nondirective counselling, the person being counselled determines the content and direction of the counselling and explores conflict and emotions at the time. While allowing empathic reflection, the counsellor does not offer advice and feedback.

COGNITIVE BEHAVIOURAL APPROACH

The cognitive behavioural approach assumes that the person would like to change and analyses situations that cause the psychological problem, so that these can be altered. Problem solving techniques, self-monitoring, anger management, relapse prevention, assertiveness training and the acquisition of social skills and modification of irrational beliefs or patterns of thought or behaviour are used. For instance, individual, group and family therapies used in the treatment of psychological symptoms and psychiatric disorders are often based on cognitive behavioural approaches.

SOCIAL NETWORK BEHAVIOUR THERAPY

Social network behaviour therapy considers the social environment as being important in the development, maintenance and resolution of problems. It maximises positive social support, which is central to the process. The therapist offers advice and feedback and thereby facilitates change in the person's social world. Behaviour is not interpreted and engagement with significant others is key in bringing about change and achieving goals.

FAMILY THERAPY

Family therapy involves attempts to understand and interpret the family dynamics in order to change the psychopathology. Psychological problems are perceived as a symptom of family dysfunction and so altering the dynamics brings about change. Family members are viewed as contributory to the problems. Behavioural techniques may be used in family therapy as well as psychodynamic techniques.

MOTIVATIONAL INTERVIEWING

Motivational interviewing aims to build motivation for change. The focus is on a nonjudgemental approach and the person's concerns and choices: it elicits strategies from the individual. Motivational enhancement directs the person to motivation for change by offering empathic feedback, advice and information and selectively reinforces certain discrepancies that emerge between current behaviour and goals, in order to enhance motivation for change. Significant others play some part in the treatment but do not have a central role. It is, by and large, a personal therapeutic situation where the individual's motivation is seen as vital. It aims to alter the decisional balance so that patients themselves direct the process of change.

Delivery of services: monitoring, review and coordination

Collaborative working with other professionals, based on a broadly based multicomponent approach is essential. Services should be designed so that leadership and management are brought together, with an awareness of the views of users and carers, the clinical realities and the evidence to date. It is vital that it is recognised that there are high levels of comorbidity of substance misuse, psychiatric disorder and many other health, educational and social problems for young women. Thus, multidisciplinary and multi-agency services need to be responsive to the real needs of the patient groups by providing the 'right' organisational culture and therapeutic environment. There is a need to provide comprehensive and accessible services for parents and children by involving mental health services with children's services at an early stage in the treatment plan.

Evidence suggests that support with housing, other health and social needs and family involvement produces a better outcome, so that inter-agency collaboration is not just of academic importance.

BREAKING THE CYCLE

Just as pregnant women, mothers and older women may be affected by their history of previous psychosocial experiences and physical health problems, the next generation may be at potential risk, arising out of the consequences of maternal or familial ill-health. Hence, the detection and management of psychological problems is an opportunity that should not be missed.

KEY POINTS

- At present, there is a rapidly accumulating evidence base in the understanding and treatment of psychological disorder.

- Treatment should follow a comprehensive assessment and be part of an overall management plan adapted to the intensity and complexity of the presenting problems.

- Emphasis must be placed on engagement and retention in services, noting that the interventions provided interact with the familial, cultural and environmental background of the woman.

- While it may not be appropriate for the obstetrician and gynaecologist to initiate treatment, women will arrive already on medication. It is necessary to assess whether there may be contraindications related to the obstetric or gynaecological condition, pregnancy in particular. Thus, there is the need to be aware of the type and range of medications available and those which are most commonly used, as well as the adverse effects and especially those in pregnant and nursing mothers.

- There are some groups of women who are at particular risk of neglect from services. Examples are very young women, older women, the socially disadvantaged, the homeless, those with a history of offending behaviour, substance misusers and those from ethnic minorities. These women may experience a great deal of difficulty in seeking support, being offered sustained help, keeping in contact with services and compliance with treatment. Since their needs are often multiple, these groups usually need additional support in the coordination and monitoring of provision. Often they feel less stigmatised by 'medical' services for physical problems. Thus, this should be used as the chance to ascertain the need for other services which may be as important, or more important, than the reason for which the woman has consulted you.

Reference

1. Lewis G, editor. *Why Mothers Die 2000–2002. The Sixth Report of the Confidential Enquiries into Maternal Deaths in the United Kingdom.* London: RCOG Press; 2004.

2 Basic science

Neuroanatomy

Although neuroanatomy, neurochemistry and neurophysiology do not fall within the day-to-day knowledge required from gynaecologists, a basic understanding is useful to understand hypothalamo-pituitary function and the effects of various steroid hormones and neuroendocrine modulators in the pathophysiology of psychological disorders. Neuroanatomy and neurophysiology are complex and only broadly relevant to the obstetric and gynaecological trainee. Although it is extremely unlikely that direct questions on knowledge of the following neuroanatomy or neurophysiology will be asked in a clinical RCOG examination, it is valuable to be aware of the terminology.

HYPOTHALAMUS

The hypothalamus is located within the ventromedial portion of the diencephalon. It is situated inferior to the thalamus and in close proximity to the pituitary gland (Figure 2.1). This brain region is important for fluid regulation, thermoregulation, food intake, reproduction, sympathetic and parasympathetic function and the control of circadian rhythms. Many of these actions are mediated through hypothalamic control of anterior and posterior pituitary function.

Hypothalamic nuclei

A nucleus refers to an aggregation of neuronal cell bodies. The major hypothalamic nuclei are the preoptic area, suprachiasmatic nucleus, supraoptic nucleus, paraventricular nucleus, ventromedial nucleus and arcuate nucleus. Each of these nuclei is involved in a specialised function (Figure 2.2).

The paraventricular nucleus produces the hypothalamic hypophysiotrophic hormones. These peptides are transported into the anterior pituitary (adenohypophysis), via a portal vessel system, where they either stimulate or inhibit the release of other hormones. Examples of these releasing hormones are thyrotrophin-releasing hormone (TRH),

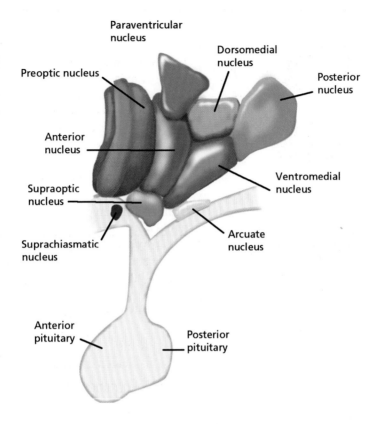

Figure 2.1 Sagittal view of the pituitary gland and its relation to the hypothalamic nuclei

which stimulates the release of thyroid-stimulating hormone (TSH) and corticotrophin-releasing hormone (CRH), which releases adreno-corticotrophic hormone (ACTH). The TSH and ACTH then act on the thyroid and adrenal glands respectively. The release of hormones from these effector organs is controlled by a positive and negative feedback loop.

The paraventricular nucleus and supraoptic nucleus contain magno-cellular neurosecretory cells that send their axons into the posterior pituitary, or neurohypophysis, where they release the peptide hormones vasopressin and oxytocin directly into the bloodstream. Vasopressin plays a major role in controlling blood pressure and maintaining blood osmolality through its vasoconstrictive and water-

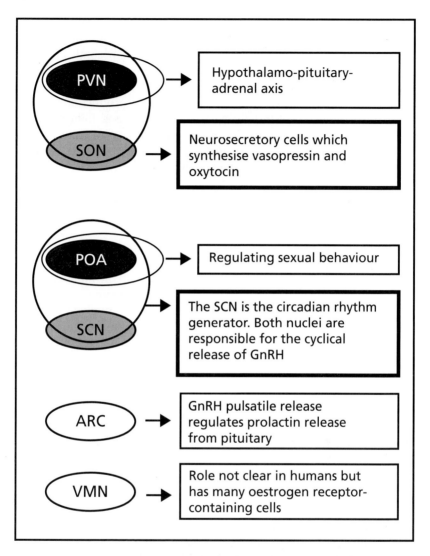

Figure 2.2 The major hypothalamic nuclei and their main functions; preoptic area (POA), suprachiasmatic nucleus (SCN), supraoptic nucleus (SON), paraventricular nucleus (PVN), ventromedial nucleus (VMN) and arcuate nucleus (ARC), gonadotrophin-releasing hormone (GnRH)

retaining characteristics. Effects of oxytocin include milk let down during lactation and uterine contraction during labour. Both hormones also modulate brain neuronal activity and can exert profound influences on behaviour.

The preoptic area, suprachiasmatic nucleus and arcuate nucleus play important roles in sexual behaviour and reproduction. The preoptic area is the circadian rhythm generator, and both the preoptic area and the suprachiasmatic nucleus work together to produce cyclical release of gonadotrophin-releasing hormone (GnRH). GnRH is important in maintaining the cyclicity inherent in female reproduction. GnRH stimulates the release of luteinising hormone (LH) and follicle-stimulating hormone (FSH). The arcuate nucleus seems to regulate gonadotrophin production through controlling the pulsatile release of GnRH. It is also important in controlling prolactin release by the anterior pituitary.

THE LIMBIC SYSTEM

The limbic system is a functionally organised group of brain regions involved in many affective behaviours (Table 2.1). There is no unanimity on which of the brain's structures make up the limbic system. It is a neural substrate for emotional experience and expression. Some of its structures (such as the hippocampus) are also involved in other complex brain processes such as memory. Through efferent and afferent pathways from and to the hypothalamaus, cerebral cortex and basal ganglia, the limbic system is able to integrate highly processed sensory and cognitive information with the autonomic and endocrine systems.

Table 2.1 The main brain regions constituting the limbic system	
Region	Function
Hippocampus	Integral to learning and memory
Amygdala	Central to perception of fear and expression of stress
Nucleus accumbens	Known as the 'reward centre' because of its crucial involvement in addictive behaviours
Periaqueductal grey	Relay station for the regulation of responses as aggression, anxiety, pain perception and sexual behaviour

Neurochemistry

THE OPIATE SYSTEM AND THE HYPOTHALAMOPITUITARY–OVARIAN AXIS

Endogenous opioid peptides control the release of LH by inhibiting the activity of hypothalamic neurones that release GnRH. In postmenopausal females, naloxone (opioid antagonist) has no effect on LH release but hormone replacement therapy (HRT) increases LH response. The release of LH is modulated by the sex steroid hormone milieu.[1]

There is evidence to suggest that oestrogen can directly affect the number and function of opioid receptors and may directly stimulate these receptors.[2,3] Moreover, cyclical administration of oestrogen-progestin to menopausal women also significantly increases serum level of beta-endorphin.[4] Therefore, the proposed beneficial effects of HRT on behaviour and mood may operate through changes in circulating opioid levels. Of course, other neuropeptide pathways may be equally important.

GONADAL STEROID HORMONES AND THE SEROTONERGIC SYSTEM

Oestrogen has mood-enhancing properties and can also increase sensitivity to serotonin, possibly by inhibiting monoamine oxidase (MAO). MAO is the enzyme responsible for the breakdown of serotonin. Progesterone also modulates serotonin; it causes increased serotonin uptake and turnover in several brain areas in rats, consequently effectively decreasing serotonin activity (Figure 2.3). Increased levels of MAO activity in depressed women have been shown to be significantly reduced by oestrogen replacement therapy.[5,6] Preliminary studies suggest that oestrogen can augment the antidepressant effect of SSRIs in perimenopausal women. This adjunctive treatment strategy seems superior to antidepressant therapy or oestrogen replacement alone.[5,7,8] However, well-designed, prospective trials are needed to evaluate the contribution of oestrogen under these circumstances.

There is also evidence that gonadal hormones are involved in regulating the expression of serotonin (5-HT) receptors. In animal studies long-term oestrogen treatment results in a decrease in 5-HT1 and an increase in 5-HT2 receptors. Mood disorders associated with puberty, menopause and during the menstrual cycle may, therefore, result from the altered distribution or function of serotonin receptor subtypes brought on by changes in the hormonal milieu.

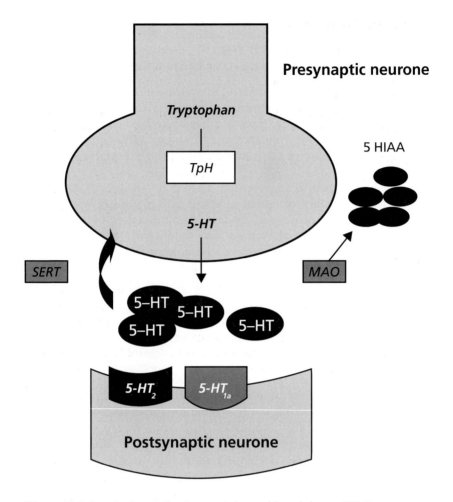

Figure 2.3 Serotonin synthesis, reuptake and breakdown; **MAO** = monoamine oxidase, **SERT** = serotonin transporter, **TpH** = tryptophan hydroxylase, **5-HT** =serotonin (5-hydroxy tryptamine), **5-HIAA** = 5 hydroxy indolacetic acid

Serotonergic dysfunction has been implicated in the aetiology of premenstrual syndrome, premenstrual dysphoric disorder (PMDD), postpartum depression and perimenopausal mood disorders.[9,10] The potential association of these steroid hormones with serotonin seems particularly relevant to mood change in premenstrual, postpartum and perimenopausal mood disturbances.

THE DOPAMINE SYSTEM

Dopamine has been shown to influence reproductive behaviour by modulating oestrogen and progesterone receptor activity.[11,12] Gonadal steroids also modulate the dopamine system and affect dopamine receptor expression.[13,14]

The effect of circulating sex steroids on dopamine receptor expression and modification may explain the gender differences observed in many psychological and neurological disorders, particularly schizophrenia and Parkinson's disease. Women tend to have a later onset of schizophrenia and the incidence of Parkinson's disease is greater in men than in women. Moreover, Alzheimer's disease appears to progress more slowly in women receiving HRT.[15] This area continues to remain controversial and unproven.

THE GABA SYSTEM

Gamma amino butyric acid (GABA) is a major inhibitory neurotransmitter in the central nervous system (CNS). It can be found in up to 30% of CNS synapses. Loss or blockade of GABA inhibition can result in increased hyper-excitability and expression of seizures.

Progesterone is converted to neuroactive steroids (5α-pregnane steroids) in the brain. Progesterone metabolites (allopregnanolone and pregnanolone) appear to have anxiolytic and hypnotic properties via GABA type A (GABA-A) agonist activity. Therefore, dysfunction in the GABA-A/neurosteroid system has been implicated in the aetiology of mood disorders and premenstrual syndrome.[16,17] Throughout reproductive life, progesterone production seems to have an influence on women's psychological health.[18] This appears to be enhanced in the period of time leading up to the menopause. Progesterone and its metabolites, such as allopregnanolone, are produced by the ovary and the adrenals and also *de novo* in the brain. Both are neurosteroids that readily cross the blood brain barrier.[19,20] They exert actions through specific receptors in the brain, affecting neuronal function and neurotransmission, thus producing their behavioural effects. Progesterone has a modulatory influence on sleep intensity and pattern.[21] Allopregnanolone is implicated in the influence of progesterone on sleep. It is a GABA-A receptor agonist, causing a rapid depression of neuronal excitability.[22–24] This may explain why women experiencing menopausal transition report an increase in depressive symptoms and impaired sleep.[25] An alternative mechanism is that the night sweats and flushes have a direct effect on sleep and depression (the domino effect) rather than the neuroendocrine mechanism.

References

1. Genazzani AR, Gastaldi M, Bidzinska B, Mercuri N, Genazzani AD, Nappi RE, *et al.* The brain as a target organ of gonadal steroids. *Psychoneuroendocrinology* 1992;17:385–90.
2. Zhou L, Hammer RP Jr. Gonadal steroid hormones upregulate medial preoptic mu-opioid receptors in the rat. *Eur J Pharmacol* 1995;278:271–4.
3. Zakon HH. The effects of steroid hormones on electrical activity of excitable cells. *Trends Neurosci* 1998;21:202–7.
4. Ortega E, Cuadros JL, Gonzalez AR, Ruiz E. Effects of estrogen-progestin replacement therapy on plasma beta-endorphin levels in menopausal women. *Biochem Mol Biol Int* 1993;29:831–6.
5. Halbreich U, Kahn LS. Role of estrogen in the aetiology and treatment of mood disorders. *CNS Drugs* 2001;15:797–817.
6. Meltzer HY. Role of serotonin in depression. *Ann N Y Acad Sci* 1990;600:486–99.
7. Liu P, He FF, Bai WP, Yu Q, Shi W, Wu YY, *et al.* Menopausal depression: comparison of hormone replacement therapy and hormone replacement therapy plus fluoxetine. *Chin Med J (Engl)* 2004;117:189–94.
8. Westlund TL, Parry BL. Does estrogen enhance the antidepressant effects of fluoxetine? *J Affect Disord* 2003;77:87–92.
9. Steiner M, Dunn EJ. The psychobiology of female-specific mood disorders. *Infertil Reprod Med Clin North Am* 1996;7:297–313.
10. Toren P, Dor J, Rehavi M, Weizman A. Hypothalamic-pituitary-ovarian axis and mood. *Biol Psychiatry* 1996;40:1051–5.
11. Apostolakis EM, Garai J, Fox C, Smith CL, Watson SJ, Clark JH, *et al.* Dopaminergic regulation of progesterone receptors: brain D5 dopamine receptors mediate induction of lordosis by D1-like agonists in rats. *J Neurosci* 1996;16:4823–34.
12. Gangolli EA, Conneely OM, O'Malley BW. Neurotransmitters activate the human estrogen receptor in a neuroblastoma cell line. *J Steroid Biochem Mol Biol* 1997;61:1–9.
13. Di Paolo T. Modulation of brain dopamine transmission by sex steroids. *Rev Neurosci* 1994;5:27–41.
14. Manzanares J, Wagner EJ, LaVigne SD, Lookingland KJ, Moore KE. Sexual differences in kappa opioid receptor-mediated regulation of tuberoinfundibular dopaminergic neurons. *Neuroendocrinology* 1992;55:301–7.
15. Asthana S, Baker LD, Craft S, Stanczyk FZ, Veith RC, Raskind MA, *et al.* High-dose estradiol improves cognition for women with AD: results of a randomized study. *Neurology* 2001;57:605–12.
16. Rapkin AJ, Morgan M, Goldman L, Brann DW, Simone D, Mahesh VB. Progesterone metabolite allopregnanolone in women with premenstrual syndrome, *Obstet Gynecol* 1997;90:709–14.
17. Romeo E, Strohle A, Spalletta G, di Michele F, Hermann B, Holsboer F, *et al.* Effects of antidepressant treatment on neuroactive steroids in major depression, *Am J Psychiatry* 1998;155:910–13.
18. Gruber CJ, Huber JC. Differential effects of progestins on the brain. *Maturitas* 2003;46 Suppl 1:S71–5.
19. Paul SM, Purdy RH. Neuroactive steroids. *FASEB J* 1992;6:2311–12.
20. Purdy RH, Morrow AL, Moore PH Jr, Paul SM. Stress-induced elevations of gamma-aminobutyric acid type A receptor-active steroids in the rat brain. *Proc Natl Acad Sci U S A* 1991;88:4553–7.
21. Gandolfo G, Scherschlicht R, Gottesmann C. Benzodiazepines promote the intermediate stage at the expense of paradoxical sleep in the rat. *Pharmacol Biochem Behav* 1994;49:921–7.
22. Bitran D, Purdy RH, Kellogg CK. Anxiolytic effect of progesterone is associated with increases in cortical allopregnanolone and GABAA receptor function. *Pharmacol Biochem Behav* 1993;45:423–8.

23. Korneyev A, Costa E. Allopregnanolone (THP) mediates anesthetic effects of progesterone in rat brain. *Horm Behav* 1996;30:37–43.
24. Picazo O, Fernandez-Guasti A. Anti-anxiety effects of progesterone and some of its reduced metabolites: an evaluation using the burying behavior test. *Brain Res* 1995;680:135–41.
25. Genazzani AR, Gambacciani M, Simoncini T, Schneider HP; International Menopause Society. "Controversial issues in climacteric medicine" series 3rd Pisa workshop "HRT in climacteric and aging brain". Pisa, Italy, 15–18 March 2003. *Maturitas* 2003;46:7–26.

3 The menarche

Introduction

Gender differences in the prevalence of mood disorders have been well documented. Prior to adolescence, the rate of depression is more or less similar in girls and boys; yet, with the onset of puberty, there is an associated increase in prevalance of depression as well as other psychiatric disorders in girls (Figure 3.1).[1,2] Puberty is also a period of social and sexual tension; these can be the precipitating factors for the development of psychological disorders such as eating disorders, anxiety, panic attacks, substance and alcohol misuse.

It is not known what proportion of the psychological change around puberty and the subsequent teens is the direct consequence of adolescence itself as opposed to the direct psychoneuroendocrine effects of previously unfamiliar cyclical hormone changes. There are many changes occurring at this period of life. It would be naïve to attribute all of the psychological changes at puberty to a single hormonal, genetic, environmental, familial or psychosocial factor and all of these must be considered.

Puberty

Puberty is the period of time during which secondary sexual characteristics are being developed. Menstruation begins and the psychosexual outlook of girls changes. The most important fact about pubertal changes is that it varies in the age of onset, time of development and order of appearance. The average age of menarche in the UK is 13 years and 95% of the population will reach it between the ages of 11 years and 15 years.[3]

Aetiological factors related to mood disorders in female adolescents

PUBERTAL STATUS

Pubertal status is defined as the current level of physical development of

(a) Age 5–10 years

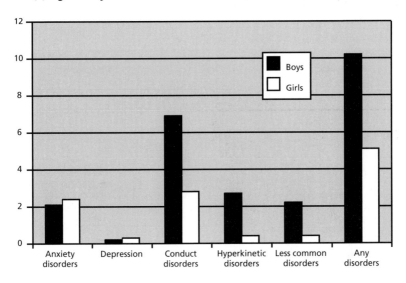

(b) Age 11–16 years

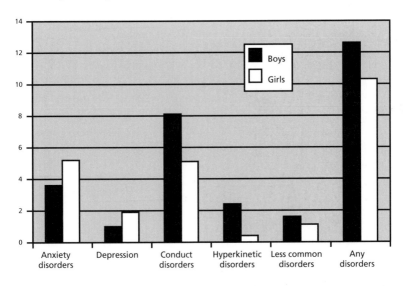

Figure 3.1 Prevalence of psychiatric disorders among boys and girls aged 5–16 years (source: Mental Health of Children and Young People in Great Britain, 2004. National Statistics; Crown copyright; (a) Age 5–10 years, (b) Age 11–16 years

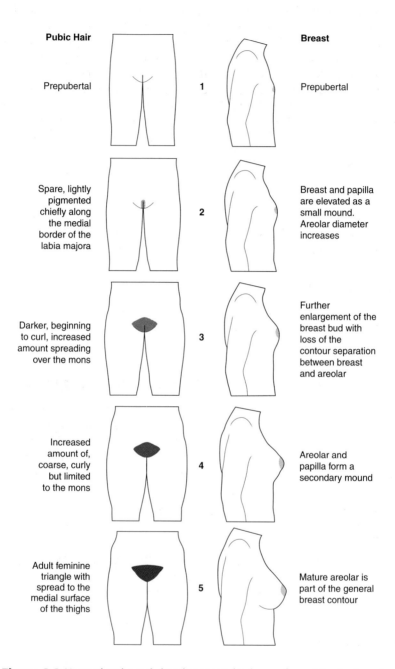

Figure 3.2 Normal pubertal development (redrawn from Marshall and Tanner 1969, with permission)

an adolescent relative to the overall process of pubertal change, usually denoted by a series of stages from pre-pubertal (stage 1) to adult (stage 5)(Figure 3.2).[4] At puberty, girls' attitudes about their physical appearance become more negative and may be closely associated with negative affect.[5,6] This contrasts sharply with the positive association in boys between increased height and muscle bulk and increased self-esteem.

Depression rates in girls (unlike boys) seem to rise significantly in mid-puberty, i.e. with the transition to Tanner stage 3.[7] Moreover, pubertal status rather than age at puberty better predicts the emergence of the sex ratio in depression rates.

PUBERTAL TIMING

This is defined as the maturation of an adolescent relative to her peers. Girls who mature earlier manifest more emotional and behavioural problems and have poorer psychological adjustment.[6]

PSYCHOSOCIAL STRESSORS

The onset of major depression in adolescence has been significantly related to experiencing a severe life event such as physical assault, childhood neglect or abuse or family illness (Figure 3.3).[8–10]

FAMILY PSYCHIATRIC HISTORY AND GENETIC FACTORS

The presence or history of maternal depression significantly increases the likelihood of depression in female children and adolescents.[11] Although it is difficult to separate genetic factors from environmental influences, there is evidence of increased heritability for depression in adolescent girls; this evidence is based on a study of pubertal twins.[9]

HORMONES AND NEUROMODULATORS

Hypothalamo-pituitary-adrenal system

Altered hypothalamic-pituitary-adrenal (HPA) system function has been observed in persons diagnosed with major depression.[12] Early physical and emotional stress in animals has also been shown to be associated with altered HPA axis function and suppression of reproductive function (including delayed puberty); similar associations have been identified in young women.[13]

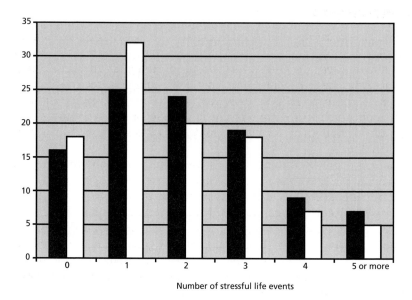

Number of stressful life events

Figure 3.3 Stressful life events by type of emotional and conduct disorder, all children, 2004 (source: Mental Health of Children and Young People in Great Britain, 2004. National Statistics; Crown copyright.

Serotonergic system

There is some evidence of the involvement of the serotonergic system in the aetiology of depressive disorders in child and adolescent depression.[14,15] Gonadal hormones seem to affect the number and function of serotonin receptors. The altered distribution or function of serotonin receptor subtypes brought on by changes in the hormonal milieu at menarche may increase vulnerability to mood disorders.

RELATIONSHIP PROBLEMS

Relationship problems could be a common cause for depression in this age group. Problems tend to occur in adolescents' relationships with their parents as well as with their peers. Depressed children and teenagers are frequently unable or reluctant to talk about their sadness. They are sometimes unable to label their feelings accurately; they instead express themselves with irritability, impatience and anger, making it difficult for their parents to offer the emotional support and guidance the child actually needs in this situation.

Management

For diagnosis, standardised criteria need to be used. The *International Classification of Diseases*, 10th edition (ICD-10) criteria for mood disorders is used throughout the world, including in the UK. Young people with mental health problems have complex needs and may require a range of services. GPs vary widely in their recognition of childhood psychiatric disorders and only refer a small proportion of disordered children to specialist child and adolescent mental health services.[16,17]

There is paucity of clinical trials assessing psychopharmacological treatment in mood disorders in adolescents. Moreover, there are concerns about the long-term safety of such medication for children and adolescents. Hence, psychotherapy is most often recommended as the first-line intervention for adolescents with mild to moderate depression.

There is little specific treatment that the gynaecologist should be offering, unless there is clearly a severe menstrually related mood disorder when psychotherapeutic or psychological interventions have been unsuccessful or considered inappropriate.

References

1. Lewinsohn PM, Rohde P, Seeley JR. Major depressive disorder in older adolescents: prevalence, risk factors and clinical implications. *Clin Psychol Rev* 1998;18:765–94.
2. Kessler RC, Walters EE. Epidemiology of DSM-IIIR major depression and minor depression among adolescents and young adults in the National Comorbidity Survey. *Depress Anxiety* 1998;7:3–14.
3. Edmonds DK. Gynaecological disorders of childhood and adolescence. In: Edmonds K, editor. *Dewhurst's Textbook of Obstetrics and Gynaecology for Postgraduates*. Oxford: Blackwell Science; 1999.
4. Tanner JM. *Growth at Adolescence*. 2nd ed. Oxford: Blackwell Scientific; 1962.
5. Brooks–Gunn J. Antecedents and consequences of variations in girls' maturational timing. *J Adolesc Health Care* 1988;9:365–73.
6. Hayward C, Killen JD, Wilson DM, Hammer LD, Litt IF, Kraemer HC, *et al.* Psychiatric risk associated with early puberty in adolescent girls. *J Am Acad Child Adolesc Psychiatry* 1997;36:255–62.
7. Angold A, Costello EJ, Worthman CM. Puberty and depression: the roles of age, pubertal status and pubertal timing. *Psychol Med* 1998;28:51–61.
8. Williamson DE, Birmaher B, Frank E, Anderson BP, Matty MK, Kupfer DJ. Nature of life events and difficulties in depressed adolescents. *J Am Acad Child Adolesc Psychiatry* 1998;37:1049–57.
9. Silberg J, Pickles A, Rutter M, Hewitt J, Simonoff E, Maes H, *et al.* The influence of genetic factors and life stress on depression among adolescent girls. *Arch Gen Psychiatry* 1999;56:225–32.
10. Weiss EL, Longhurst JG, Mazure CM. Childhood sexual abuse as a risk factor for depression in women: psychosocial and neuro-biological correlates. *Am J Psychiatry* 1999;156:816–28.
11. Shiner RI., Marmorstein NR. Family environments of adolescents with lifetime depression: associations with maternal depression history. *J Am Acad Child Adolesc Psychiatry* 1998;37:1152–60.

12. Holsboer F, Lauer CJ, Schreiber W, Krieg JC. Altered hypothalamic-pituitary-adrenocortical regulation in healthy subjects at high familial risk for affective disorders. *Neuroendocrinology* 1995;62:340–7.
13. De Bellis MD, Putnam FW. The psychobiology of childhood maltreatment. *Child Adolesc Psychiatric Clin North Am* 1994;3:663–77.
14. Hughes CW, Petty F, Sheikha S, Kramer CL. Whole-blood serotonin in children and adolescents with mood and behavior disorders. *Psychiatry Res* 1996;65:79–95.
15. Sallee FR, Vrindavanam NS, Deas-Nesmith D, Odom AM, Carson SW, Sethuraman G. Parenteral clomipramine challenge in depressed adolescents: mood and neuroendocrine response. *Biol Psychiatry* 1998;44:562–7.
16. Garralda E. Child and adolescent psychiatry in general practice. *Aust N Z J Psychiatry* 2001;35:308–14.
17. Maughan B, Brock A, Ladva G. Mental health. In: Office for National Statistics. *The Health of Children and Young People*. London: ONS; 2004.

4   The menstrual cycle

Introduction

The menstrual cycle commences with the maturation of the hypothalamo-pituitary-ovarian axis. At menarche each ovary contains about 300 000 primordial follicles. Once maturation has commenced, follicles proceed to either maturation or atresia; the latter is the fate of the majority. The high luteal phase levels of progesterone produced by the corpus luteum resulting from ovulation are blamed for most of the physical and behavioural premenstrual symptoms. At least one premenstrual symptom occurs in 95% of women during the reproductive age. The physical symptoms (mastalgia, bloatedness) have also been attributed to progesterone through induced fluid retention. However, there is now much evidence to suggest that this is not true.

Premenstrual syndrome

Premenstrual syndrome (PMS) is a psychological and somatic disorder of unknown aetiology. Hormonal and other, possibly neuroendocrine, factors probably contribute.[1,2] There has been a reluctance, until relatively recently, to accept PMS as a serious condition. This has arisen because of a general failure to distinguish true PMS from the milder physiological premenstrual symptoms occurring in the normal menstrual cycle of the majority of women.

DEFINITION

A woman can be diagnosed as having PMS if she complains of recurrent psychological or somatic symptoms (often both), occurring specifically during the luteal phase of the menstrual cycle and resolving by the end of menstruation. These symptoms must be so severe that they disrupt the woman's normal functioning, quality of life and interpersonal relationships. Symptoms must have occurred in at least four of the previous six cycles. The character of the symptoms is less important than their timing and severity in that, as well as occurring in the luteal phase, they must be absent in the time between the end of menstruation and ovulation. This is a key diagnostic feature.

Table 4.1. Research criteria for premenstrual dysphoric disorder

A. In most menstrual cycles during the past year, five (or more) of the following symptoms were present for most of the time during the last week of the luteal phase, began to remit within a few days after the onset of the follicular phase and were absent in the week post-menses, with at least one of the symptoms being either (1), (2), (3), or (4):

  (1) Markedly depressed mood, feelings of hopelessness or self-deprecating thoughts.

  (2) Marked anxiety, tension, feelings of being 'keyed up', or 'on edge'.

  (3) Marked affective lability (e.g. feeling suddenly sad or tearful or increased sensitivity to rejection).

  (4) Persistent and marked anger or irritability or increased interpersonal conflicts.

  (5) Decreased interest in usual activities (e.g. work, school, friends, hobbies).

  (6) Subjective sense of difficulty in concentrating.

  (7) Lethargy, easy fatiguability or marked lack of energy.

  (8) Marked change in appetite, overeating or specific food cravings.

  (9) Hypersomnia or insomnia.

  (10) A subjective sense of being overwhelmed or out of control.

  (11) Other physical symptoms, such as breast tenderness or swelling, headaches, joint or muscle pain, a sensation of bloating, weight gain.

Note: In menstruating women, the luteal phase corresponds to the period between ovulation and the onset of menses and the follicular phase begins with menses. In non-menstruating women (e.g. those who have had a hysterectomy), the timing of luteal and follicular phases may require measurement of circulating reproductive hormones.

B. The disturbance markedly interferes with work or school or with usual social activities and relationships with others (e.g. avoidance of social activities, decreased productivity and efficiency at work or school).

C. The disturbance is not merely an exacerbation of the symptoms of another disorder, such as major depressive disorder, panic disorder, dysthymic disorder or a personality disorder (although it may be superimposed on any of these disorders).

D. Criteria A, B, and C must be confirmed by prospective daily ratings during at least two consecutive symptomatic cycles (the diagnosis may be made provisionally prior to this confirmation).

Reproduced with permission from *Diagnostic and Statistical Manual of Mental Disorders*, 4th ed. © American Psychiatric Association.

PREMENSTRUAL DYSPHORIC DISORDER

There is now a trend, especially with psychiatrically trained clinicians, to redefine PMS based upon the criteria of the fourth version of the *Diagnostic and Statistical Manual of Mental Health* (DSM-IV). It was termed late-luteal-phase dysphoric disorder (LLPDD) in DSM-III, and is now premenstrual dysphoric disorder (PMDD) under DSM-IV. Table 4.1 shows the criteria for a DSM-IV PMDD diagnosis. It is important to be clear what is meant by the terms PMDD and PMS, as current literature often uses them interchangeably. PMDD is the extreme, predominantly psychological end of the PMS spectrum. It is mainly used by American psychiatrists.

PMDD is defined in the DSM-IV as outlined in Table 4.1 being present for most of the last week of the luteal phase and remitting within a few days after the onset of the follicular phase. At least one of the symptoms must be from the cluster of PMDD-defining symptoms. The disturbance caused by the symptoms must interfere markedly with work, school or usual social activities and relationships with others. The disturbance must not be an exacerbation of another psychiatric disorder such as major depression disorder, panic disorder, dysthymic disorder or personality disorder.

AETIOLOGY OF PMS/PMDD

The definitive aetiology of PMS/PMDD is still unknown, although it appears to be directly related to the ovarian cycle trigger. There is a range of theories proposed as possible causes.

Hormonal disturbances

It has long been suggested that fluctuation in mood may be related to ovarian hormone imbalance.[3] Research has produced data that could support theories of oestrogen excess, progesterone deficiency, oestrogen/progesterone imbalance and progesterone excess. None of these theories has been confirmed and, thus, factors other than differences in the levels of individual hormones must be important, since it is increasingly apparent that women with PMS/PMDD have normal levels of ovarian hormones. Interactions with other endocrine, biochemical or neurotransmitter systems must operate. Alternatively, differences in progesterone receptor status may be relevant.

PMS/PMDD and the ovarian cycle

A link with ovarian hormone changes, particularly progesterone, seems likely, since the temporal relationship between progesterone production and symptoms is so close. Ablation of the ovarian endocrine cycle by oophorectomy or by the administration of analogues of GnRH is associated with the parallel elimination of PMS symptoms.[4] Furthermore, in women whose ovarian cycles have ceased (due to the menopause or bilateral oophorectomy) and who subsequently receive HRT, a significant percentage redevelop PMS symptoms during the progestogen phase of therapy.[5]

In a pilot study, women with severe PMS who had undergone hysterectomy and bilateral salpingo-oophorectomy were recruited to assess the effects of hormone replacement on their PMS symptoms.[6] During oestrogen-only replacement therapy they remained asymptomatic; when progesterone was administered, PMS symptoms recurred, demonstrating fairly clearly that they remained sensitive to the effects of progesterone.

Serotonin

The knowledge of serotonin involvement in depression has been extended into PMS research. Low serotonin levels in red cells and platelets have been demonstrated in women with PMS.[7] It has been proposed that this serotonin deficiency enhances sensitivity to progesterone.[2] Selective serotonin reuptake inhibitors (SSRIs), such as fluoxetine and sertraline, increase synaptic serotonin and have been shown to be extremely efficacious treatments for severe PMS/PMDD.[8] This gives further indirect support to the involvement of serotonin in PMS aetiology. Vitamin B6 (pyridoxine) is a cofactor in the final step in the synthesis of serotonin and dopamine from tryptophan. However, no data have yet demonstrated consistent abnormalities either of brain amine synthesis or deficiency of vitamin B6.

Other neurotransmitters may have relevance to PMS, for example GABA, dopamine and acetylcholine, although research data are less convincing for these in comparison to that for beta-endorphin and serotonin.

Endorphins

Chuong et al.[9] have demonstrated diminished luteal-phase levels of beta-endorphin in women with PMS. Symptoms such as anxiety, food craving and physical discomfort have been associated with a significant premenstrual decline in beta-endorphin levels.[10]

Allopregnanolone deficiency

Investigations of the metabolites of progesterone suggest that women with PMS have lower levels of the progesterone metabolite allopregnanolone in the luteal phase of the cycle.[2] This is a plausible theory because allopregnanolone has a sedative and anxiolytic effect through its GABA-ergic activity. Deficiency of allopregnanolone may, therefore, give rise to PMS symptoms.

DIAGNOSIS

PMS may be confused with many other disorders and the diagnosis of PMS itself may be difficult. Underlying psychopathology can be prospectively quantified and excluded using established questionnaires. These must be completed only in the follicular phase of the cycle. Cyclical symptoms are most precisely rated daily using visual analogue scales or menstrual distress questionnaires (Figure 4.1). These should be used prospectively for two cycles. Quality-of-life health surveys have been used to measure the degree to which the woman's life is disrupted. These symptoms can be recorded and analysed manually or, more conveniently, using a handheld computer which incorporates the above questionnaires as well as a series of visual analogue scales. Such a computer system is capable of recording and transferring these measures to a computer database producing 'clinician-friendly' graphic displays of the severity and the timing of the symptoms in relation to the menstrual cycle.

In some difficult cases it may be of value to use a GnRH analogue depot for 3 months to distinguish to what degree the ovarian cycle contributes to symptoms.

There are currently no biochemical tests for PMS. However, blood tests may be considered to exclude other disorders such as menopause, polycystic ovary syndrome, hyper- and hypothyroidism and anaemia.

The physical examination of a woman with PMS will make little contribution to her diagnosis, but the exclusion of disorders that may mimic somatic symptoms (pelvic pain and abdominal bloatedness) must be stressed. Reassurance that there is no breast, cervical or pelvic cancer is of particular value and, of course, women should not receive hormonal therapy without such an examination.

Steiner et al.[11] reported a tool that could be used to screen for PMS/PMDD (the premenstrual symptoms screening tool, PSST). The PSST reflects and 'translates' categorical DSM-IV criteria for PMDD into a rating scale with degrees of severity. They concluded in their study that this tool is less time-consuming and more practical than two cycles of prospective charting and that it is an effective screening tool and an important starting point for further assessment.

Day of Cycle	1	2	3	4	5	6	7	8	9	10	11	12	13	14	15	16	17	18	19	20	21	22	23	24	25	26	27	28	29	30	31	32	33	34
Day of Month																																		
Irritability																																		
Mood swings																																		
Depression																																		
Hostility																																		
Sadness																																		
Negative thoughts																																		
Bloating																																		
Breast pain																																		
Appetite changes																																		
Carbohydrate cravings																																		
Hot flushes																																		
Insomnia																																		
Headache																																		
Fatigue																																		
Confusion																																		
Poor concentration																																		
Social withdrawal																																		
Hyperphagia																																		
Arguing																																		
Decreased Interest																																		

Day #1 is the first day of cycle. (ie first day of menses)
Use one chart for each menstrual cycle
Luteal Phase and thus, ovulation occurs 14 days before menses

Severity Code: 0=none, 1=mild, 2=moderate, 3=severe

Figure 4.1 Calendar of premenstrual experience (COPE) for the daily rating of menstrual symptoms

MANAGEMENT

PMS does not seem to be caused by an endocrine imbalance *per se*. However, it appears that there is increased sensitivity to the normal circulating level of ovarian hormones, particularly progesterone, secondary to a neuroendocrine disturbance, probably serotonin deficiency. If this is factually correct, an approach to therapy using this hypothesis does seem practical and effective. Accordingly, approaches to treatment fall into two broad strategies:

- suppression of ovulation (Table 4.2)
- correction of the neuroendocrine anomaly (Table 4.3).

Table 4.2 Suppression of ovulation	
Preparation/ treatment	**Use/evidence**
Progesterone and progestogens	There is not enough evidence to support effectiveness. A systematic review of progesterone and progestogen versus placebo found no improvement in overall premenstrual symptoms.[12] In general, progesterone has been given cyclically with no attempt to suppress ovulation
Oestrogen	Studies suggest that oestrogenic ovarian suppression eliminates PMS.[13,14] Oestrogen can be used in the form of patches (100–200 micrograms), implants (50–100 mg) or gel. The latter seems to be effective only for premenstrual migraine. Progestogens, necessarily used to protect the uterus from the untoward effects of unopposed oestrogen, may reintroduce PMS. To avoid this systemic effect, progestogen may be used locally (levonorgestrel-releasing intrauterine system). Clinical experience and early non-blind studies suggest this to be very effective
Danazol	Ovulation suppression can be achieved by danazol. It is no longer licensed for the treatment of PMS because of concerns of potential masculinising effects, lipid change and possibly ovarian cancer. Luteal-phase danazol seems to be effective for premenstrual breast pain only and without a significant high rate of short-term adverse effects[15,16]
GnRH analogues (GnRHa)	The use of GnRHa in PMS is limited because significant trabecular bone loss occurs after only 6 months of analogue treatment. The use of GnRH analogues in PMS serves the following purposes: ■ It allows us to determine what proportion of symptoms is of ovarian endocrine origin. ■ It pinpoints which women with severe PMS would benefit from bilateral oophorectomy should they be undergoing hysterectomy for gynaecological pathology.

- It offers short-term therapy of 6 months in particular circumstances.
- It may be useful for women in whom oestrogens are contraindicated and who are shortly to reach the menopause.

A meta-analysis has clearly demonstrated the efficacy of GnRHa and the effect is not diminished by addback therapy, particularly when tibolone is used, which prevents menopausal adverse effects and may permit prolonged therapy[17]

Oral contraceptives	It would be anticipated that the combined oral contraceptive pill (COCP), which acts predominantly by suppressing ovulation, would also eliminate PMS. Surprisingly the limited trials do not support this. Probably the reintroduction of a new oestrogen/progestogen cycle is the reason for this. Continuous COCP ought to prevent this but it (anecdotally) does not seem to be universally effective. Surprisingly, there are no trials. A COCP containing drospirenone has shown possible benefit in a limited number of studies.[20] This new progestogen has anti-mineralocorticoid effects and there is a theoretical reason why this 'spironolactone-like' effect may improve physical symptoms. Developments are awaited.
Hysterectomy and bilateral salpingo-oophorectomy	Hysterectomy with bilateral oophorectomy is curative but rarely justified; it may be indicated if there are coexisting gynaecological problems. Women who will benefit must first be identified as being treatable in this fashion following a positive goserelin* test. Surgery must be followed by oestrogen replacement, which should be unopposed
Laparoscopic bilateral oophorectomy	Simplifying surgery by retaining the uterus and removing only the ovaries laparoscopically significantly reduces the invasiveness of the surgery. However, the remaining presence of the uterus demands endometrial protection. Systemic progestogens will risk restimulating the PMS symptoms. These patients were premenopausal prior to surgery and so should receive oestrogen replacement or tibolone until at least the age of 50 years. A goserelin/ leuprorelin plus tibolone test would normally be undertaken prior to surgery and so tibolone may be continued thereafter; alternatively, oestradiol with a levonorgestrel intrauterine system may be appropriate. Total abdominal hysterectomy and bilateral salpingo-oophorectomy must also be considered as a last resort and only used on the patient's insistence

* The use of GnRH agonist analogues such as goserelin or leuprorelin produces a temporary menopause like state. The absence of ovulation and thus a luteal phase progesterone, not surprisingly, eliminates all the symptoms of PMS. The resulting menopause-like symptoms can be prevented with tibolone (addback) without restimulation of PMS. This mimics the effect of removing the uterus and ovaries (followed by HRT) and should predict the eventual result of surgery. It is not possible to conduct a placebo-controlled trial where such major surgery is involved and so evidence for this 'test' is limited. There are, however, robust studies that demonstrate the elimination of symptoms using GnRH and addback

Table 4.3 Correction of the neuroendocrine anomaly

Preparation	Use/evidence
Selective serotonin reuptake inhibitors	There is strong evidence that SSRIs are effective in treating physical as well as behavioural PMS symptoms. SSRIs used in trials include fluoxetine, sertraline, citalopram, fluvoxamine and paroxetine.[8] Common adverse effects were headache, nervousness, insomnia, drowsiness/fatigue, sexual dysfunction and gastrointestinal disturbances. Fluoxetine is no longer licensed for PMDD in Europe but it is in the USA
Other antidepressants and anxiolytics	Antidepressants (bupropion, clomipramine, nortriptyline and desipramine), beta-blockers (atenolol and propranolol), anxiolytics (alprazolam and buspirone) have been assessed in adequately controlled trials. These demonstrated benefit for one or more symptoms of PMS, although some women stop treatment because of adverse effects. Additionally, these drugs appear to be less effective than SSRIs
Vitamin B6	Vitamin B6 is a co-factor in the final stages of neurotransmitter synthesis, particularly of serotonin and dopamine, from tryptophan. In practice, many women will have self-prescribed vitamin B6 before consulting their doctor. Results of a meta-analysis are equivocal and point to the inadequacy of the published studies[18]

MANAGEMENT OF PMDD

A panel of European researchers discussed PMDD and the algorithm for its management was proposed. This may help with individual patients (Figure 4.2).[19]

PREMENSTRUAL EXACERBATION

Some disorders are exacerbated during the premenstrual period. Examples of such disorders include affective disorders, anxiety disorders, substance misuse, allergies, eating disorders, asthma, migraine and seizures. Women with PME constitute one of the largest groups of women with premenstrual problems. These women are not considered to have premenstrual syndrome because they do not have a week free of symptoms. Daily ratings and even clinical interviews can be helpful in these cases. Management depends on the nature and degree of the underlying disorder. The gynaecologist's role in these situations is complementary to the role of the physician or psychiatrist who is managing the primary disorder.

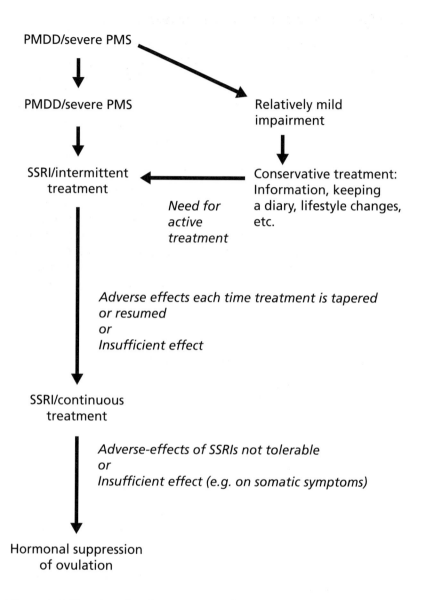

Figure 4.2 Flowchart for the treatment plan in premenstrual dysphoric disorder (PMDD) and severe premenstrual syndrome (PMS); SSRI = selective serotonin reuptake inhibitor (modified from Eriksson E, *et al.*)[19]

Functional hypothalamic amenorrhoea

Another probable psychological condition related to menstrual-cycle disturbance is amenorrhoea. This condition was previously referred to as idiopathic or psychogenic amenorrhoea in the psychiatric literature. It is a diagnosis of exclusion. The disorder can be viewed as a functional reduction in GnRH secretion, which results in reduced pituitary secretion of gonadotrophins and subsequent ovarian quiescence. However, the peripheral and central signals that contribute to the initiation and maintenance of the inhibition of GnRH in the disorder are poorly understood. The current standard practice, other than observation, is to offer pharmacological interventions, such as oral contraceptives and hormone replacement if fertility is not desired and pharmacological ovulation induction if fertility is desired. However, pharmacological intervention alone does not lead to spontaneous recovery and cannot be expected to ameliorate the stress-induced alterations in central neurotransmission and hypothalamic function. Moreover, the direct impact on the psychological symptoms themselves has not been systematically evaluated.

References

1. O'Brien PMS. Helping women with premenstrual syndrome. *BMJ* 1993;307:1471–5.
2. Rapkin AJ, Morgan M, Goldman L, Brann DW, Simone D, Mahesh VB. Progesterone metabolite allopregnanolone in women with premenstrual syndrome. *Obstet Gynecol* 1997;90:709–14.
3. Dalton K. *The Premenstrual Syndrome and Progesterone Therapy*. London: Heinemann; 1977.
4. Hussain SY, Massil JH, Matta WH, Shaw RW, O'Brien PMS. Buserelin in premenstrual syndrome. *Gynaecol Endocrinol* 1992;6:57–64.
5. Hammarbäck S, Backstrom T, Hoist J, von Schoultz B, Lyrenas S. Cyclical mood changes as in the premenstrual tension syndrome using sequential oestrogen-progestagen postmenopausal replacement therapy. *Acta Obstet Gynecol Scand* 1985;64:393–7.
6. Henshaw C, Foreman D, Belcher J, Cox J, O'Brien S. Can one induce premenstrual symptomatology in women with prior hysterectomy and bilateral oophorectomy? *J Psychosom Obstet Gynaecol* 1996;17:21–8.
7. Rapkin AJ. The role of serotonin in premenstrual syndrome. *Clin Obstet Gynecol* 1992;35:629–36.
8. Dimmock PW, Wyatt KM, Jones PW, O'Brien PM. Efficacy of selective serotonin-reuptake inhibitors in premenstrual syndrome: a systematic review. *Lancet* 2000;356:1131-6.
9. Chuong CJ, Coulam CB, Kao PC, Bergstralh EJ, Go VL. Neuropeptide levels in premenstrual syndrome. *Fertil Steril* 1985;44:760–5.
10. Giannini AJ, Melemis SM, Martin DM, Folts DJ. Symptoms of premenstrual syndrome as a function of beta-endorphin: two subtypes. *Prog Neuropsychopharmacol Biol Psychiatry* 1994;18:321–7.
11. Steiner M, Macdougall M, Brown E. The premenstrual symptoms screening tool (PSST) for clinicians. *Arch Womens Ment Health* 2003;6:203–9.
12. Wyatt K, Dimmock P, Jones P, Obhrai M, O'Brien PMS. Efficacy of progesterone

and progestogens in management of premenstrual syndrome: systematic review. *BMJ* 2001;323:776–80.

13. Watson NR, Studd JW, Savvas M, Garnett T, Baber RJ. Treatment of severe premenstrual syndrome with oestradiol patches and cyclical oral norethisterone. *Lancet* 1989;2:730–2.

14. de Lignieres B, Vincens M, Mauvais-Jarvis P, Mas JL, Touboul PJ, Bousser MG. Prevention of menstrual migraine by percutaneous oestradiol. *BMJ* 1986;293:1540.

15. Sarno AP Jr, Miller EJ Jr, Lundblad EG. Premenstrual syndrome: beneficial effects of periodic, low-dose danazol. *Obstet Gynecol* 1987;70:33–6.

16. O'Brien PMS, Abukhalil IEH. Randomised controlled trial of the management of premenstrual syndrome and premenstrual mastalgia using luteal phase only danazol. *Am J Obstet Gynecol* 1999;180:18–23.

17. Wyatt KM, Dimmock PW, Ismail KMK, Jones PW, O'Brien PMS. The effectiveness of GnRHa with and without 'add-back' therapy in treating premenstrual syndrome: a meta analysis. *BJOG* 2004;111:585–93.

18. Wyatt KM, Dimmock PW, Jones PW, O'Brien PMS. Vitamin B6 therapy: a systematic review of its efficacy in premenstrual syndrome. *BMJ* 1999;318:1375–81.

19. Eriksson E, Endicott J, Andersch B, Angst J, Demyttenaere K, Facchinetti F, *et al.* New perspectives on the treatment of premenstrual syndrome and premenstrual dysphoric disorder. *Arch Women Ment Health* 2002;4:111–19.

20. Freeman EW, Kroll R, Rapkin A, Pearlstein T, Brown C, Parsey K, *et al.* Evaluation of a unique oral contraceptive in the treatment of premenstrual dysphoric disorder. *J Womens Health Gend Based Med* 2001;10:561–9.

5 Psychological aspects of infertility and its management

Introduction

Parenthood is believed to be one of the major role transitions in adult life for both men and women. Thus, fertility difficulties and the associated, invasive investigations and treatment are significant causes of psychological stress. Some couples respond to this life event with relative ease, whereas others experience intense personal and interpersonal distress.

In general, women who are part of an infertile couple show higher distress. For women, infertility results in a greater loss of identity, in more pronounced feelings of failure and reduced competence, and in higher anxiety and depression levels.[1-4] Women are also more likely to avoid children, pregnant women and other reminders of the fertile world.[5,6] The man's response to infertility closely approximates the woman's but only when the cause of the infertility has been attributed to a male factor.

Whether or not it is treated, infertility can produce a variety of psychological reactions. Responses depend upon personality attributes, including adaptability, cultural expectations, support systems, knowledge about reproductive processes and the attitudes of the involved clinicians.

Effect of fertility treatment on stress, anxiety and depression

Women who undergo infertility treatment experience a loss of privacy as they cope with hospital and laboratory personnel. The sense of intimacy that reinforces marriage and mutuality may be challenged when sex and procreation are separated by technology. The change in the purpose of sexual intercourse and self-doubt about performance could be a cause of sexual dysfunction.[7,8] Also, couples and subfertility specialists have been observed to frequently overestimate the likelihood of treatment success, which often results in violated expectations.

In a desire to increase the chances of conception the transfer of multiple embryos can have deleterious psychological consequences, especially if it results in high-order multiple pregnancy, because of the associated increased risks of congenital abnormality, premature delivery and handicap. Further complexity arises where consideration is given to 'selective' fetal reduction.

It is not surprising that these treatments will create different levels of stress in both men and women. A 1-year comparative study of couples undergoing assisted reproductive treatment demonstrated that, in general, treatment-related distress and levels of depression were higher for women than for men.[9]

There are discrepancies in the reported rates of depression and anxiety in relation to fertility treatment. There is also some evidence that, even after successful infertility treatment, there is increased risk for postnatal depression and post-traumatic stress disorder in the postpartum period.[10]

Greater psychological stress has been demonstrated in women with non-anatomical infertility than in those with an anatomical cause.[11] This finding might be consistent with the hypothesis that psychosocial stress contributes to the aetiology of some forms of infertility. An alternative explanation could be that suffering from unexplained infertility could be more stressful than suffering from an identifiable anatomical cause for the infertility.

Effect of stress, anxiety and depression on fertility

The effect of stress, anxiety and depression on fertility or the outcome of infertility treatment remains a matter of debate. Some epidemiological studies suggest a link between depression and subfertility.[12] In a prospective study examining the influence of depression levels and coping on *in vitro* fertilisation outcome in women, Demyttenaere *et al.*[13] reported that expression of negative emotions predicted depression levels and outcome in *in vitro* fertilisation. Other investigators did not confirm this.[14,15]

Counselling

Psychological support services should be available for all individuals and couples undergoing active evaluation and intervention for infertility. The Human Fertilisation and Embryology Authority (HFEA) code of practice requires that all infertility units provide counselling facilities to be available for patients. In most cases, counsellors are participants of the multidisciplinary team. Counsellors, in addition to providing more structured therapy, offer women the time to 'think aloud'. This is often useful in guiding the woman through the maze of considerations, which is an important requisite in their decision making. In general, there is accumulating evidence of the positive effect of counselling in assisted conception treatment.[16]

References

1. Olshansky EF. Identity of self as infertile: an example of theory-generating research. *ANS Adv Nurs Sci* 1987;9:54–63.
2. Valentine D. Psychological impact of infertility: identifying issues and needs. *Soc Work Health Care* 1987;11:61–9.
3. Mahlstedt PP, Macduff S, Bernstein J. Emotional factors and the in-vitro-fertilization and embryo transfer process. *J In Vitro Fert Embryo Transf* 1987;4:232–6.
4. Wright J, Duchesne C, Sabourin S, Bissonnette F, Benoit J, Girard Y. Psychosocial distress and infertility: men and women respond differently. *Fertil Steril* 1991;55:100–8.
5. Greil AL, Leitko TA, Porter KL. Infertility: his and hers. *Gender Society* 1988;2:172–99.
6. Berg BJ, Wilson JF, Weingartner PJ. Psychological sequelae of infertility treatment: the role of gender and sex-role identification. *Soc Sci Med* 1991;33:1071–80.
7. Drake TS, Grunert GM. A cyclic pattern of sexual dysfunction in the infertility investigation. *Fertil Steril* 1979;32:542–5.
8. Saleh RA, Ranga GM, Raina R, Nelson DR, Agarwal A. Sexual dysfunction in men undergoing infertility evaluation: a cohort observational study. *Fertil Steril* 2003;79:909–12.
9. Beutel M, Kupfer J, Kirchmeyer P, Kehde S, Kohn FM, Schroeder-Printzen I, *et al.* Treatment-related stresses and depression in couples undergoing assisted reproductive treatment by IVF or ICSI. *Andrologia* 1999;31:27–35.
10. Bartlik B, Greene K, Graf M, Sharma G, Melnick H. Examining PTSD as a complication of infertility. *Medscape Womens Health* 1997;2:1.
11. Wasser SK, Sewail G, Soules MR. Psychosocial stress as a cause of infertility. *Fertil Steril* 1993;59:685–9.
12. Grodstein F, Goldman MB, Ryan L, Cramer DW. Self-reported use of pharmaceuticals and primary ovulatory infertility. *Epidemiology* 1993;4:151–6.
13. Demyttenaere K, Bonte L, Gheldof M, Vervaeke M, Meuleman C, Vanderschuerem D, *et al.* Coping style and depression level influence outcome in *in vitro* fertilization. *Fertil Steril* 1998;69:1026–33.
14. Harlow CR, Fahy UM, Talbot WM, Wardle PG, Hull MG. Stress and stress-related hormones during in-vitro fertilization treatment. *Hum Reprod* 1996;11:274–9.
15. Milad MP, Klock SC, Moses S, Chatterton R. Stress and anxiety do not result in pregnancy wastage. *Hum Reprod* 1998;13:2296–300.
16. Emery M, Beran MD, Darwiche J, Oppizzi L, Joris V, Capel R, *et al.* Results from a prospective, randomized, controlled study evaluating the acceptability and effects of routine pre-IVF counselling. *Hum Reprod* 2003;18:2647–53.

6   Pregnancy and the puerperium

Pregnancy loss

The break of the attachment to the unborn child and the resulting grief and bereavement is an appropriate starting point for understanding the psychological reactions to pregnancy loss.

MISCARRIAGE

Miscarriage is the most common complication of pregnancy. There is consensus in the literature that 'distress' commonly follows spontaneous miscarriage.[1] However, there is considerable disagreement between studies regarding the intensity and nature of this distress (for example, grief versus depression), its duration and what factors predict its intensity and duration. Some authors have argued that health professionals devalue the significance of miscarriage for the women involved, underestimate its emotional impact and fail to provide much-needed support.[1] In contrast, others state that 'the overzealous may interfere with the healthy resilience that enables most people to get over an early miscarriage without becoming psychiatrically disturbed'.[2]

Many authors have advocated that women should be routinely assessed after miscarriage and offered counselling. In a randomised controlled trial assessing debriefing after miscarriage, Lee et al.[3] were unable to demonstrate any positive effect upon emotional adaptation. Debriefing can even have negative effects for some couples by interfering with their adaptive suppression and distraction. The beneficial component of debriefing seems to be the detailed explanation of events. This can, however, only be provided by the obstetric staff involved and is unavailable from the counsellor.

It seems apparent that a substantial number of women do experience adverse reactions, which commonly extend over several months. The extent to which these equate with grief as opposed to depression is unclear. A minority of women, probably less than 10%, appear to suffer more enduring adverse reactions extending beyond 6 months.[4]

Although it might be assumed that grief and emotional turmoil would be related to gestational age, this assumption is not supported by observations.[5]

Unlike infertility, which can continue indefinitely, pregnancy loss is a defined event with an end. Acute reactions to an isolated miscarriage or perinatal loss such as blame, guilt, anger, and denial gradually lead to acceptance and resolution. A single miscarriage does not predict poor future reproductive performance. Recurrent pregnancy loss carries a less favourable pregnancy and psychological prognosis and resembles infertility in its chronicity and sense of lost potential.

TERMINATION OF PREGNANCY

There are conflicting reports in the literature about the psychological sequelae of termination of pregnancy. These reports require more cautious interpretation for several reasons.[4] The intense controversy and debate surrounding legal, moral and ethical aspects of this issue have sometimes introduced bias and lack of scientific objectivity. Inadequate attention to the heterogeneous nature of the procedures considered (first- versus second-trimester termination, legal versus illegal abortion, termination of a wanted versus an unwanted pregnancy, termination of a wanted pregnancy for fetal abnormalities versus psychosocial pressures, termination which conflicts with strongly held religious or moral values versus one which does not).

A large study carried out under the auspices of the Royal College of General Practitioners compared 6410 women who had termination of pregnancy with 6151 women who did not. The rates of psychiatric disorders were not significantly different between the two cohorts. In both groups, significantly elevated rates were found in women with a past history of psychiatric illness. However, even in women with no previous history of psychiatric illness, deliberate self-harm was more common in the cohort who had undergone termination.[6]

Risk factors for adverse sequelae include past psychiatric illness, termination of a wanted pregnancy (for medical or psychosocial reasons) and a lack of social support.[7,8] The presence of one or more of these risk factors should not be a contraindication to termination but rather an indication for more thorough monitoring and supportive intervention both prior to and after termination.[9]

LATE PREGNANCY LOSS

The grief and bereavement model facilitates the understanding and the management of women suffering pregnancy loss. However, this can sometimes lead to the overlooking of severe psychiatric illness in bereaved woman. The first task of the clinician is to exclude severe psychiatric disorders such as major depression, psychosis or post-traumatic stress disorder. The events surrounding the death, including the behaviours and attitudes of the obstetric and neonatal staff, are critically important in influencing the psychological outcome.[10]

In grief therapy, the pregnancy experience should be explored as well as the reactions of significant others. In subsequent sessions, the events occurring at the time of loss are covered including the perceived reaction of staff and family. Anger and guilt are frequent components of the reaction to pregnancy loss. Guilt is one of the most difficult emotions to work with in this type of therapy. Prolonged grief can happen in women who have not adequately dealt with anger and/or grief. Chronic grief is more difficult to treat.[4]

Pseudocyesis

Pseudocyesis is the development of the classic symptoms of pregnancy (amenorrhoea, nausea, breast enlargement and pigmentation, abdominal distension, and, even, labour pains) in a non-pregnant woman. Pseudocyesis demonstrates the ability of the psyche to dominate the soma, probably via central input at the level of the hypothalamus. Predisposing psychological processes are thought to include a pathological wish for and fear of pregnancy or conflict regarding gender, sexuality or childbearing and a grief reaction to lost potential following a miscarriage, tubal ligation or hysterectomy. Psychotherapy is recommended during or after a presentation of pseudocyesis to evaluate and treat the underlying psychological dysfunction.

Postpartum psychiatric disorders

Various investigators have argued that postpartum mental illness consists of a group of psychiatric disorders that are specifically related to pregnancy and childbirth and therefore exists as a distinct diagnostic entity. However, evidence suggests that affective illness that emerges during the puerperium does not differ significantly from affective illness occurring in women at other times. This opinion is reflected in DSM-IV, which includes postpartum psychiatric illness as a subtype of either bipolar disorder or major depressive disorder.

Postpartum psychiatric illnesses have a long-lasting effect on the woman, the marital relationship and the child's emotional, social and cognitive development.[11] The likelihood of a woman experiencing a depressive episode in the postpartum period is higher in women with a family history and/or personal history of depressive disturbance. Obstetric difficulties appear to be irrelevant in both puerperal psychosis and postnatal depression. There is a three-fold increase in the relative risk of depression in the first five postnatal weeks.[12] Postpartum psychiatric illnesses are classified into five groups:[13]

- maternity blues

- pure postpartum depression

- previous history of major and minor depression

- postpartum psychosis

- comorbid emergence of postpartum depression.

MATERNITY BLUES

It was not until the 1960s that Pitt first described an 'atypical' depression (later called 'maternity blues') that affected mothers soon after childbirth.[14] Maternity blues are relatively common, affecting 50–80% of postnatal women. They begin on the second or third postnatal day and should start to remit by second week.[15] The clinical significance of the blues is that 25% of these women will go on to develop depression.

As postpartum blues are usually mild in severity and resolve spontaneously, no specific treatment other than support and reassurance is indicated. However, the woman should be instructed to contact her obstetrician, midwife or primary care provider if the symptoms persist for longer than 2 weeks, to ensure the early identification of a more severe affective illness. Women with histories of psychiatric illness, particularly previous postpartum depression, should be monitored more closely, as they are at higher risk for significant puerperal illness. Identification of women at high risk is considered desirable in the antenatal period.

POSTPARTUM DEPRESSION

'Pure' postnatal depression is seen in 10–12% of women, usually within the first 4 weeks after delivery.[16-18] The onset of depression is early, rapid and often severe enough to require therapy. Relapse rates, in future pregnancies, have been estimated at 24–40%.[19] Postpartum depression may affect women with evidence of previous episodes of major or minor depression, although it may not have been diagnosed.

In co-morbid emergence of postpartum depression, an anxiety disorder that has been present for a long time (often mild and not diagnosed) is primary. Panic attacks, generalised anxiety or obsessive-compulsive disorder are evident from the woman's history. In the postpartum period, the anxiety disorder worsens and is followed by the emergence of depression. These women should always be investigated to exclude an underlying medical disorder, particularly Hashimoto's thyroiditis.

Severe postpartum depression is easily recognised but milder or more insidious forms of depressive illness are frequently missed. Since it is difficult to predict reliably which women in the general population are likely to develop puerperal illness, some advise screening of all women for depression during the postpartum period. The standard postpartum obstetric visit at 6 weeks and subsequent paediatric appointments are ideal times to screen for postpartum depressive illness. The Edinburgh Postnatal Depression Scale (EPDS) is a ten-item, self-rated question-naire (Appendix 6.1) that has been used extensively for the detection of postpartum depression and has demonstrated satisfactory sensitivity and specificity in women during the postpartum period.

The EPDS was developed at health centres in Livingston and Edinburgh. It consists of ten short statements. The mother underlines the response closest to how she has been feeling during the previous week. Most mothers complete the scale without difficulty in less than 5 minutes. The initial validation study showed that mothers who scored above a threshold 12/13 were likely to be suffering from a depressive illness of varying severity. The scale indicates how the mother has felt during the previous week and, in doubtful cases, it may be usefully repeated after 2 weeks. The scale will not detect mothers with anxiety neuroses, phobias or personality disorders.

The mother is asked to underline the response that comes closest to how she has been feeling in the previous 7 days. All ten items must be completed. Care should be taken to avoid the possibility of the mother discussing her answers with others. The mother should complete the scale herself, unless she has limited English or has difficulty with reading. The EPDS may be used at 6–8 weeks to screen postnatal women. The child health clinic, postnatal check-up or a home visit may provide suitable opportunities for its completion.

In postpartum depression, hospitalisation is warranted if the mother is assessed to be a danger to herself or to her baby and there is an inadequate family support structure for the mother.

Pharmacotherapy using anxiolytic and antidepressant medications backed up by supportive psychotherapy are important in managing the condition. Fluoxetine and the other SSRIs are ideal first-line agents because they are anxiolytic, generally non-sedating and well tolerated.

Cognitive behavioural therapy may also be useful in this setting. There is evidence that short-term cognitive behavioural therapy is as effective as treatment with fluoxetine in women with postpartum depression.[20] There seem to be distinct advantages in managing women with postpartum depression in specific multi-professional 'mother and baby' units. One of the standards set by the National Service Framework for Children, Young People and Maternity Services is that women should have easy access to supportive, high-quality maternity services, designed around their individual needs and those of their babies. It is recommended in this document that healthcare professionals should be competent in identifying and addressing mental health problems for women during or after pregnancy and that local perinatal psychiatric services are available for women who need them.

POSTPARTUM PSYCHOSIS

Postpartum psychosis occurs following 0.05–0.10% of births.[21] Psychosis presents acutely in the first 2–4 weeks postpartum with symptoms resembling mania with delusions, hallucinations, agitation and confusion. It requires hospital admission and aggressive pharmacological management. A careful history usually reveals onset within the first few days after delivery. Prominent symptoms at that time are restlessness and sleeplessness, which could be misinterpreted as excitement about the new baby. Postpartum psychosis carries a high risk of recurrence (more than 90%) in future pregnancies.[18]

Postpartum psychosis is a dangerous illness that carries a risk of infanticide and suicide. It is a psychiatric emergency that requires inpatient treatment. Mood stabilising medications (lithium, valproic acid or carbamazepine) should be started immediately along with antipsychotic agents. Breastfeeding is typically avoided in women treated with lithium, as it is secreted at significant levels into the breast milk and may cause neonatal toxicity. Electroconvulsive therapy is well tolerated and rapidly effective. Failure to treat puerperal psychosis aggressively places both the mother and infant at increased risk of harm.

AETIOLOGY OF POSTPARTUM PSYCHIATRIC ILLNESSES

The aetiology of postpartum psychiatric disorders is likely to be heterogeneous and the interaction between biological, psychological and social factors is extremely complex. Consistent endocrine differences have not been found between women who develop postnatal depression and those who do not.[22] However, failure to demonstrate systemic evidence of hormone deficiencies does not exclude sex hormones as aetiological factors. Peripheral hormone levels need not correspond with brain levels, nor are they necessarily an index of brain receptor numbers and affinity. It is possible that a susceptible subpopulation of women experiences mental disorders as a result of the progesterone or oestrogen withdrawal.[13]

ROLE OF OESTROGEN IN POSTPARTUM PSYCHIATRIC DISORDERS

It has been suggested that oestrogen therapy is effective in treating postpartum depression and in reducing the risk of recurrence of puerperal depression and postpartum psychosis.[23] However, high-dose oestrogen may add to the risk of thromboembolism at a time when the chances of this complication are at their highest. Because of this risk, as well as endometrial hyperplasia and inhibition of lactation, it is unlikely that oestrogen will be investigated further in the management of postpartum psychiatric disorders.[24–26]

Psychopharmocological treatment during pregnancy

Therapeutic benefits gained from psychopharmacological treatment must be weighed against potential risks to the fetus. Fetal risks from exposure can include abnormal fetal growth, teratogenic effects, withdrawal symptoms and even fetal death. In addition to fetal risks, medication effects can intensify somatic symptoms of pregnancy; for example, decreased gastrointestinal emptying and constipation.

Only a small proportion of birth defects are caused by medications taken by the mother in pregnancy. Where possible, medication should be avoided in the first 12 weeks and for longer if practicable. Medication should be prescribed if risks of, for example, psychotic illness, outweigh the risks of taking medication. Almost all psychotropic drugs cross the placenta and are excreted in breast milk, albeit in small quantities.

Consultation with specialist clinicians is advised for all women needing psychotropic medication who are pregnant or breastfeeding. In general, the psychiatrist will evaluate the severity of a psychiatric disorder and thus the balance of risk and benefit. This risk–benefit assessment needs careful consideration. In women with long-term mental illness necessitating psychotropic medication, one should aim to avoid combination therapies, stop nonessential medications (e.g. benzodiazepines) and reduce essential drugs. There is rarely a valid reason to stop essential drug treatment during pregnancy. Conventional antipsychotics are relatively safe for the fetus, so women taking atypical antipsychotics should be switched to conventional antipsychotics before they conceive.

GENERAL APPROACH TO TREATMENT IN PREGNANCY

- Counselling and dose/drug adjustment should be done prior to attempts at conception.
- Try to avoid combination therapies in view of their greater potential of teratogenicity.
- Select the drug with most favourable risk–benefit profile.
- Consider non-pharmacological alternatives.
- In the majority of cases, women who become pregnant while on medication need to be maintained on medication.
- Maintenance strategies should involve dosage reduction and regular review of adverse effects.
- Discontinuation of mood stabilisers in pregnancy should take place only when absolutely necessary and be followed by frequent monitoring.
- Management should be collaborative between the psychiatric team, obstetricians and midwives.
- Adequate daily folate intake is required with anticonvulsants.

Modified from Kohen (2004)[26]

References

1. Frost M, Condon JT. The psychological sequelae of miscarriage: a critical review of the literature. *Aust N Z J Psychiatry* 1996;30:54–62.
2. Bourne S, Lewis E. Perinatal bereavement. *BMJ* 1991;302:1167–8.
3. Lee C, Slade P, Lygo V. The influence of psychological debriefing on emotional adaptation in women following early miscarriage: a preliminary study. *Br J Med Psychol* 1996;69:47–58.
4. Condon JT. Pregnancy loss. In: Steiner M, Yonkers KA, Eriksson E, editors. *Mood Disorders in Women*. London: Martin Dunitz; 2000. p. 353–69.
5. Adler NE, David HP, Major BN, Roth SH, Rusoo NF, Wyatt GE. Psychological responses after abortion. *Science* 1990;248:41–4.
6. Gilchrist AC, Hannaford PC, Frank P, Kay CR. Termination of pregnancy and psychiatric morbidity. *Br J Psychiatry* 1995;167:243–8.
7. Romans-Clarkson SE. Psychological sequelae of induced abortion. *Aust N Z J Psychiatry* 1989;23:555–65.
8. Zolese G, Blacker CV. The psychological complications of therapeutic abortion. *Br J Psychiatry* 1992;160:742–9.
9. Tietze C. Contraceptive practice in the context of non-restrictive abortion law: age specific pregnancy rates in New York City, 1971–1973. *Fam Plann Perspect* 1975;7:197–202.
10. Condon JT. Predisposition to psychological complications after stillbirth: a case report. *Obstet Gynecol* 1987;70:495–7.
11. Weinberg MK, Tronick EZ. The impact of maternal psychiatric illness on infant development. *J Clin Psychiatry* 1998;59:53–61.
12. Cox JL, Murray D, Chapman G. A controlled study of the onset, duration and prevalence of postnatal depression. *Br J Psychiatry* 1993;163:27–31.

13. Sichel DA. Postpartum psychiatric disorders. In Steiner M, Yonkers KA, Eriksson E, editors. Mood disorders in women. London: Martin Dunitz; 2000. 313–28.
14. Pitt B. 'Atypical' depression following childbirth. *Br J Psychiatry* 1968;114:1325–35.
15. Kendell RE, McGuire RJ, Connor Y, Cox JL. Mood changes in the first three weeks after childbirth. *Affect Disord* 1981;3:317–26.
16. Kumar R, Robson KM. A prospective study of emotional disorders in child bearing women. *Br J Psychiatry* 1984;144:35–47.
17. O'Hara MW, Neunaber DJ, Zekoski EM. Prospective study of postpartum depression: prevalence, course and predictive factors. *J Abnorm Psychol* 1984;93:158–71.
18. Kendell RE, Chalmers JC, Platz C. Epidemiology of puerperal psychosis. *Br J Psychiatry* 1987;150:662–73.
19. Davidson J, Robertson E. A follow-up study of postpartum illness. *Acta Psychiatr Scand* 1985;71:451–7.
20. Appleby L, Warner R, Whitton A, Faragher B. A controlled study of fluoxetine and cognitive-behavioural counselling in the treatment of postnatal depression. *BMJ* 1997;314:932–6.
21. Brockington I. *Motherhood and Mental Health*. Oxford: Oxford University Press; 1996.
22. Wilcox DL, Yovich JL, McColm SC, Phillips JM. Progesterone, cortisol and oestradiol 17β in the initiation of human parturition: Partitioning between free and bound hormone in plasma. *Br J Obstet Gynaecol* 1985;92:65–71.
23. Gregoire AJP, Kumar R, Everitt B, Henderson AF, Studd JW. Transdermal oestrogen for the treatment of severe postnatal depression. *Lancet* 1996;347:930–3.
24. Sichel DA, Cohen LS, Robertson LM, Ruttenberg A, Rosenbaum JF. Prophylactic oestrogen in recurrent postpartum affective disorder. *Biol Psychiatry* 1995;38:814–18.
25. Lawrie TA, Herxheimer A, Dalton K. Oestrogens and progestogens for preventing and treating postnatal depression. *Cochrane Database Syst Rev* 2000;(4).
26. Kohen D. Psychotropic medications in pregnancy. *Adv Psychiatr Treatment* 2004;10:59–66.
27. Cox JL, Holden JM, Sagovsky R. Detection of postnatal depression: development of the 10-item Edinburgh Postnatal Depression Scale. *Br J Psychiatry* 1987;150:782–6.

Appendix 6.1.

Edinburgh Postnatal Depression Scale

(JL Cox, JM Holden, R Sagovsky, Department of Psychiatry, University of Edinburgh)

Name:

Address:

Baby's age:

As you have recently had a baby, we would like to know how you are feeling. Please UNDERLINE the answer which comes closest to how you have felt IN THE PAST 7 DAYS, not just how you feel today.

In the past 7 days:

1. **I HAVE BEEN ABLE TO LAUGH AND SEE THE FUNNY SIDE OF THINGS**
   As much as I always could.
   Not quite so much now.
   Definitely not so much now.
   Not at all.

2. **I HAVE LOOKED FORWARD WITH ENJOYMENT TO THINGS**
   As much as I ever did.
   Rather less than I used to.
   Definitely less than I used to.
   Hardly at all.

3. **I HAVE BLAMED MYSELF UNNECESSARILY WHEN THINGS WENT WRONG**
   Yes, most of the time.
   Yes, some of the time.
   Not very often.
   No, never.

4. **I HAVE BEEN ANXIOUS OR WORRIED FOR NO GOOD REASON**
No, not at all.
Hardly ever.
Yes, sometimes.
Yes, very often.

5. **I HAVE FELT SCARED OR PANICKY FOR NO VERY GOOD REASON**
Yes, quite a lot.
Yes, sometimes.
No, not much.
No, not at all.

6. **THINGS HAVE BEEN GETTING ON TOP OF ME**
Yes, most of the time I haven't been able to cope at all
Yes, sometimes I haven't been coping as well as usual
No, most of the time I have coped quite well
No, I have been coping as well as ever

7. **I HAVE BEEN SO UNHAPPY THAT I HAVE HAD DIFFICULTY SLEEPING**
Yes, most of the time.
Yes, sometimes.
Not very often.
No, not at all.

8. **I HAVE FELT SAD OR MISERABLE**
Yes, most of the time.
Yes, quite often.
Not very often.
No, not at all.

9. **I HAVE BEEN SO UNHAPPY THAT I HAVE BEEN CRYING**
Yes, most of the time.
Yes, quite often.
Only occasionally.
No, never.

10. **THE THOUGHT OF HARMING MYSELF HAS OCCURRED TO ME**
Yes, quite often.
Sometimes.
Hardly ever.
Never.

Response categories are scored 0, 1, 2, and 3 according to increased severity of the symptom.

Questions 3, 5, 6, 7, 8, 9, 10 are reverse scored (i.e., 3, 2, 1 and 0). The total score is calculated by adding together the scores for each of the ten items. A score of 12+ indicates the likelihood of depression, but not its severity. The EPDS score is designed to assist, no replace, clinical judgement.

Source
Cox JL, Holden JM, Sagovsky R. Detection of postnatal depression: development of the 10-item Edinburgh Postnatal Depression Scale. *Br J Psychiatry* 1987;150:782–6.

7 Eating Disorders

Anorexia nervosa

Anorexia nervosa is characterised by a refusal to maintain weight at or above a minimally normal weight (less than 85% of expected weight for age and height, or body mass index (BMI) less than 17.5 kg/m^2) or a failure to show the expected weight gain during growth. In assocation with this, there is often an intense fear of gaining weight, perceived body image, preoccupation with weight, denial of the current low weight and its adverse impact on health, and amenorrhoea. Two subtypes of anorexia nervosa: binge–purge and restricting, have been defined. Appendix 7.1 lists the diagnostic criteria for anorexia nervosa according to the fourth edition of the *Diagnostic and Statistical Manual of Mental Disorders.*[1]

INVESTIGATIONS

The following investigations are recommended in women with anorexia nervosa:

- erythrocyte sedimentation rate (ESR) is usually low in this condition; hence, this test can be somewhat useful in differentiating anorexia nervosa from other medical conditions causing anorexia

- electrocardiogram (ECG) is important to assess for the impact of low potassium and starvation on the heart

- computed tomography or magnetic resonance imaging to exclude the presence of cerebral tumours

- endocrine status (thyroid function and other pituitary tests)

- stool and urine tests for laxative abuse might also be useful for women suspected of such abuse

- bone density studies can be useful to further assess the physical impact of the woman's eating disorder.

COMPLICATIONS OF ANOREXIA NERVOSA

Consequences can be severe and life threatening. In a 10-year follow-up study, death occurred in approximately 7.4% of diagnosed cases.[2] Sufferers are at risk of cardiac arrest secondary to electrolyte disturbances. The severe starvation state can lead to endocrinological aberrations, which may reinforce the dieting behaviour. This can also lead to early-onset osteoporosis secondary to decreased oestrogen secretion. There is no good evidence, however, about the effects of oestrogen treatment on fracture rates in people with anorexia.[3]

MANAGEMENT OF ANOREXIA NERVOSA

The severity of illness will determine the intensity of treatment required for the anorexia nervosa patient. Treatment levels can range from an inpatient specialised eating disorder unit to a partial hospitalisation or day programme to outpatient care, depending on the weight, medical status and other psychiatric co-morbidity of the patient. The aims of treatment are to restore physical health (weight within the normal range, regular menstruation and normal bone mass); restore normal patterns of eating and attitudes towards weight and shape and treat psychiatric co-morbidity (such as depression, anxiety, obsessive compulsive disorder); and to reduce the impact of the illness on social functioning and quality of life.

The most widely used measure of outcome is the Morgan Russell scale, which includes nutritional status, menstrual function, mental state and sexual and social adjustment.[4]

Pharmacotherapy and cognitive behavioural therapy

As with many psychiatric disorders, pharmacotherapy can be used in conjunction with cognitive behavioural therapy. Antidepressants are frequently used because of the high levels of co-morbidity between anorexia nervosa, depression and obsessive–compulsive disorder. However, Treasure and Schmidt[3] found insufficient evidence from three small RCTs concerning the effects of selective serotonin reuptake inhibitors compared with placebo or no treatment in people with anorexia. They also found no evidence of benefit with amitriptyline compared with placebo.

Medical management

Medical management requires weight restoration, nutritional rehabilitation, rehydration and correction of serum electrolytes. Inpatient hospitalisation should include daily monitoring of weight, food, calorie intake and urine output. Patients should be monitored closely for attempts to vomit. Outpatients should be weighed weekly in the clinician's office, with periodic physical examinations and measurement of serum electrolytes if the patient is purging. There is limited evidence that zinc may improve daily weight gain compared with placebo in people managed in an inpatient setting.[5]

Family therapy

A family analysis should be done on all women with anorexia nervosa who are living with their families. On the basis of this analysis, a clinical judgement can be made as to what type of family therapy or counselling is advisable.

Oestrogen treatment for prevention of fractures

In a systematic review conducted by Treasure and Schmidt,[3] there were no RCTs or systematic reviews on the effects of oestrogen treatment on fracture rates in people with anorexia nervosa. Two small RCTs found no significant difference between oestrogen and placebo or no treatment in bone mineral density in people with anorexia nervosa.[3]

Bulimia nervosa

Bulimia nervosa is an intense preoccupation with body weight and shape, with regular episodes of uncontrolled overeating of large amounts of food associated with use of extreme methods to counteract the feared effects of overeating. If a person also meets the diagnostic criteria for anorexia nervosa, then the diagnosis of anorexia nervosa takes precedence.[1] Bulimia nervosa can be difficult to identify because of extreme secrecy about binge eating and purgative behaviour. Weight may be normal but there is often a history of anorexia nervosa or restrictive dieting. Some people alternate between anorexia nervosa and bulimia nervosa. The DSM-IV criteria for the diagnosis of bulimia nervosa are listed in Appendix 7.1.

COMPLICATIONS OF BULIMIA NERVOSA

Complications may include increased risk of dental caries due to enamel erosion on the teeth from vomiting, swollen parotid glands and tears in the oesophagus. These patients can also suffer from dependence on laxatives and are also at risk for cardiac arrest from electrolyte imbalance. The mortality rate for bulimia nervosa is 2.4%.

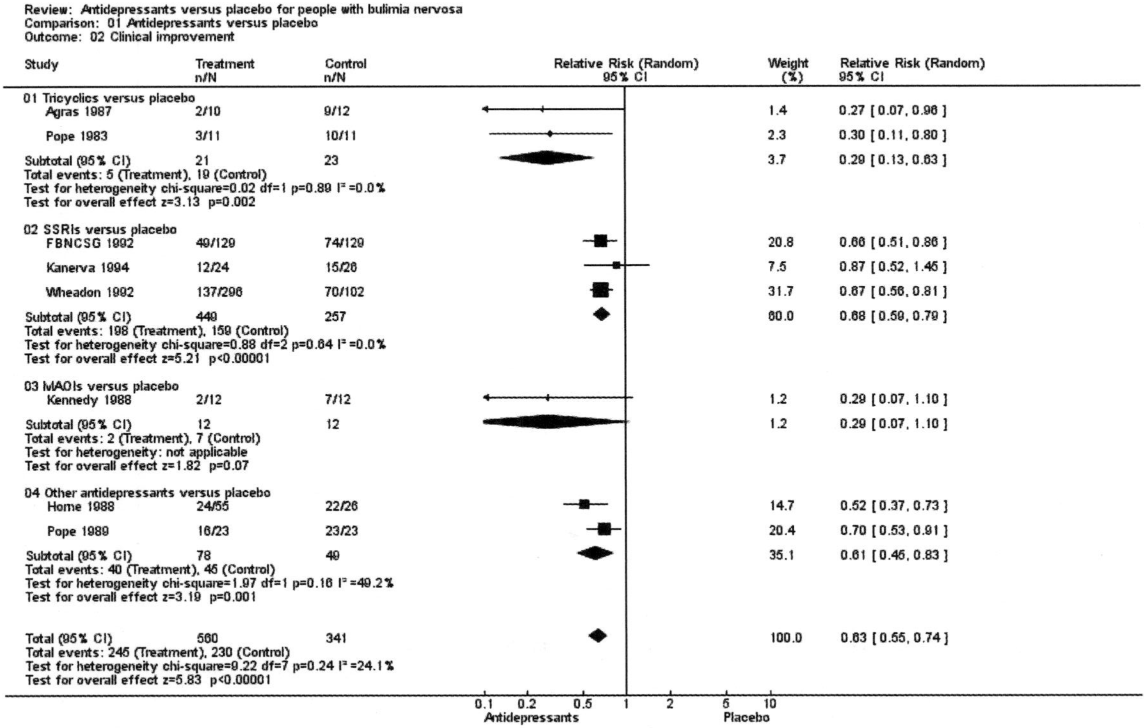

Figure 7.1 Therapeutic effectiveness of antidepressants in Bulimia nervosa (reproduced with permission from The Cochrane Library)[7]

MANAGEMENT OF BULIMIA NERVOSA

One systematic review found that cognitive behavioural therapy compared with other psychotherapies improved abstinence from binge eating and depression scores at the end of treatment.[6] In a systematic review of the published literature, Bacaltchuk and Hay[7] found strong evidence for reduction in bulimic symptoms with tricyclic antidepressants, monoamine oxidase inhibitors and fluoxetine (Figure 7.1).

Obesity and mood disorders

The obese individual has been stereotyped as being jolly and good humoured. However, for many their obesity is a consequence of chronic emotional distress. Moreover, psychological stress may promote excessive food intake not only among the obese but among those with normal weight as well. If such stress is chronic, sufficient weight will be gained to cause obesity. Psychological stress may also promote extremely rapid weight gain if it results in binge eating.

Many obese individuals consider mood disorders responsible for their inability to control their eating behaviour. Disinhibition is the inability to control food intake when experiencing negative affect. This does not only include the impulsive excessive eating of many obese individuals but also of women suffering from PMS, women with seasonal affective disorders (SAD) and individuals undergoing nicotine withdrawal. PMS and SAD generate intense cravings for carbohydrate-rich diet that may last throughout the postovulatory weeks of each menstrual cycle or from late autumn until early spring each year, respectively.

It seems that the choice of a carbohydrate-rich diet in association with the dysphoric state has a neurochemical basis.[8] Serotonin synthesis and release increase after carbohydrate intake, because of an insulin-mediated increase in the brain levels of tryptophan, the amino acid precursor of serotonin. Thus, it appears that the disinhibited obese eater is seeking to ameliorate anger, depression and tension by consuming a sweet or starchy food; this will consequently lead to obesity. When assessing women who are obese, non-psychological causes should also be considered such as Cushing's disease and polycystic ovary syndrome.

References

1. *Diagnostic and Statistical Manual of Mental Disorders*. 4th ed. Washington DC: American Psychiatric Association; 1994.
2. Crow S, Praus B, Thuras P. Mortality from eating disorders: a 5- to 10-year record linkage study. *Int J Eat Disord* 1999;26:97–101.
3. Treasure J, Schmidt U. Anorexia nervosa. *Clin Evid* 2003;9:986–96.
4. Morgan HG, Russell GF. Value of family background and clinical features as

predictors of long-term outcome in anorexia nervosa: four-year follow-up study of 41 patients. *Psychol Med* 1975;5:355–71.

5. Birmingham CL, Goldner EM, Bakan R. Controlled trial of zinc supplementation in anorexia nervosa. *Int J Eat Disord* 1994;15:251–5.
6. Hay PJ, Bacaltchuk J. Psychotherapy for bulimia nervosa and binging. *Cochrane Database Syst Rev* 2003;(1).
7. Bacaltchuk J, Hay P. Antidepressants versus placebo for people with bulimia nervosa. *Cochrane Database Syst Rev* 2003;(4): CD003391. doi: 10.1002/14651858.CD003391.
8. Wurtman R, Wurtman J. Brain serotonin, carbohydrate-craving, obesity and depression. In: Filippini GA, Costa CV, Bertazzo A, editors. *Recent Advances in Tryptophan Research: Tryptophan and Serotonin Pathways*. New York: Kluwer Academic Publishers; 1996. p. 35–41.

Appendix 7.1 DSM-IV Diagnostic criteria

Anorexia nervosa

A. Refusal to maintain body weight at or above a minimally normal weight for age and height (e.g., weight loss leading to maintenance of body weight less than 85% of that expected; or failure to make expected weight gain during period of growth, leading to body weight less than 85% of that expected).

B. Intense fear of gaining weight or becoming fat, even though underweight.

C. Disturbance in the way in which one's body weight or shape is experienced; undue influence of body weight or shape on self-evaluation, or denial of the seriousness of the current low body weight.

D. In postmenarchal females, amenorrhoea, i.e., the absence of at least three consecutive menstrual cycles. (A woman is considered to have amenorrhoea if her periods occur only following hormone, e.g., estrogen, administration.)

Specify type:

Restricting type: During the current episode of anorexia nervosa, the person has not regularly engaged in binge eating or purging behaviour (i.e., self-induced vomiting or the misuse of laxatives, diuretics, or enemas).

Binge eating/purging type: During the current episode of anorexia nervosa, the person has regularly engaged in binge eating or purging behaviour (i.e., self-induced vomiting or the misuse of laxatives, diuretics, or enemas).

Bulimia nervosa

A. Recurrent episodes of binge eating. An episode of binge eating is characterised by both of the following:
   (1) eating, in a discrete period of time (e.g., within any 2-hour period), an amount of food that is definitely larger than most people would eat during a similar period of time and under similar circumstances.
   (2) a sense of lack of control over eating during the episode (e.g., a feeling that one cannot stop eating or control what or how much one is eating).

B. Recurrent inappropriate compensatory behaviour in order to prevent weight gain, such as self-induced vomiting; misuse of laxatives, diuretics, enemas, or other medications; fasting; or excessive exercise.

C. The binge eating and inappropriate compensatory behaviours both occur, on average, at least twice a week for 3 months.

D. Self-evaluation is unduly influenced by body shape and weight.

E. The disturbance does not occur exclusively during episodes of anorexia nervosa.

Specify type:

Purging type: during the current episode of bulimia nervosa, the person has regularly engaged in self-induced vomiting or the misuse of laxatives, diuretics, or enemas.

Nonpurging type: during the current episode of bulimia nervosa, the person has used other inappropriate compensatory behaviours, such as fasting or excessive exercise, but has not regularly engaged in self-induced vomiting or the misuse of laxatives, diuretics, or enemas.

Reproduced with permission from American Psychiatric Association *Diagnostic and Statistical Manual of Mental Disorders*, 4th ed. © American Psychiatric Association.

8 Menopause and perimenopause

Introduction

It is estimated that approximately 35% of women will seek medical treatment for symptoms associated with the menopause.[1] The complaints most commonly noted by women include hot flushes, sweats, muscle and joint pain, headaches, weight gain, decreased libido, fatigue, insomnia, low mood and irritability.[2]

Definitions

The World Health Organization defines the menopause as 'the permanent cessation of menstruation resulting from loss of ovarian follicular activity'. The average age in Western women is 51 years. The perimenopause is defined as the period of time immediately before menopause when endocrinological, biological and clinical features of approaching menopause commence, until the first year after the menopause. The postmenopause is defined as dating from the time of menopause, although the exact date of the menopause cannot be determined until after a period of 12 months of spontaneous amenorrhoea has been observed.[3] Surgical menopause occurs as a result of bilateral oophorectomy, mostly at the time of hysterectomy.

Mood disorders and the menopause

Longitudinal studies have failed to demonstrate an increase in frequency of major depression or severe mood changes in relation to the transition.[4,5] Some studies, however, suggest that milder mood changes, expressed as decreased wellbeing, are more common after the menopause than before; data in this field are not consistent.[4,6–11]

Aetiology of perimenopausal and menopausal mood disorders

FLUCTUATION IN OESTROGEN LEVELS

Although genetic and psychological factors influence mood disorders during the perimenopause, periods of hormonal fluctuation or instabilities occurring during that period may precipitate the first onset or exacerbate the pre-existing risk of affective symptoms among vulnerable women.[12]

Oestrogen increases the activity of noradrenaline in the brain, thus, mimicking monoamine oxidase (MAO) inhibitor effect, resulting in higher levels of both serotonin and catecholamines. Increased levels of MAO activity in depressed women have been shown to be significantly reduced by oestrogen replacement therapy.[12]

HYPOTHYROIDISM

The incidence of hypothyroidism increases around the menopausal transition. Thyroid immune disease has been demonstrated to be an independent risk factor for depression in perimenopausal women, the incidence of which increases with age. Hypothyroidism also produces symptoms that can mimic those of perimenopause, such as fatigue, weight gain and mood change. It has been proposed that women experiencing mood disorder during the perimenopause should have their thyroid function tested.[13,14]

DECLINING ANDROGENS

There is a gradual decline in ovarian testosterone production from the age of 30 years. During the menopause testosterone levels decline to approximately 50% of the level produced in the early 20s. This decline is followed by a subsequent increase in the ovarian synthesis of androgens and a fall in sex hormone binding globulin (SHBG), leading to restoration of premenopausal levels several years after the menopause. There is also a negative correlation between age and androstenedione in women of 40–60 years of age.[27–29] Symptoms of androgen insufficiency include a decreased sense of wellbeing, dysphoria, blunted motivation, persistent unexplained fatigue, decreased energy, and decreased libido, sexual receptivity and pleasure. Other possible features related to androgen deficiency are the reduction in bone mass, decreased muscle strength and changes in cognition and memory.[15] Thus, there is evidence of potentially positive effects of androgens on overall wellbeing, mood, sexual function and bone health.[16] These effects probably augment the effect of oestrogen.[17]

Other nonhormonal known risk factors for mood changes include the stress of aging, changing body figure and changes in women's responsibilities within families, careers and communities around this period of their lives.

Hormone replacement therapy and psychological symptoms

The instability of oestrogen may influence the dysphoric and physical symptoms leading up to the menopause.[17,18] It seems that longer exposure to this hormonal fluctuation triggers a higher incidence of depression.[19] It would appear that mood disorders in the perimenopause respond to the effects of administered oestradiol, although it remains uncertain whether oestrogen has specific antidepressant properties. The contribution of oestrogens to psychological health is controversial. A meta-analysis of the effect of HRT upon depressed mood found that oestrogen treatment of menopausal women had a moderate to large benefit on mood, compared with control or placebo conditions.[20] That review found a greater effect among perimenopausal than among postmenopausal women. According to this meta-analysis, women who were treated for longer than 8 months exhibited the greatest improvement. In addition, the effect was larger for naturally versus surgically induced menopause. However, in another qualitative review, the benefits of oestrogen treatment appeared to be more consistent in surgically menopausal women.[21]

There is a possibility that psychological benefits of HRT may occur secondary to the relief of vasomotor symptoms (with insomnia) and a reduction in vaginal dryness. These findings suggest that mood enhancement in symptomatic women treated with HRT is more likely due to a 'domino effect' rather than a direct psychotropic or placebo effect, even though it is well known that there are direct effects of oestrogen on the central nervous system. A randomised study of oestrogen replacement therapy for depression in perimenopausal women also suggested indirectly that sleep disturbance by hot flushes is not the mechanism by which depression occurs in perimenopausal women as oestrogen improved depression equally in women with or without vasomotor symptoms.[22] In view of this conflicting evidence, this area remains controversial.

Morris and Rymer reviewed the published literature for evidence of the effect of oestrogen on psychological symptoms.[23] They found no RCTs of oestrogen treatment in women with clinically proven pure depression. They identified one systematic review of the effects of oestrogen on cognitive function in postmenopausal women and in women with Alzheimer's disease, which reported that studies were too weak to allow reliable conclusions to be drawn.[24] An additional cross-over RCT found a significant reduction in subjective sleep problems compared with placebo.[25] They identified four RCTs, all of which found significant improvement in quality of life among women treated with oestrogen compared with baseline or placebo.[26-29]

Hormone replacement therapy and libido

The underlying mechanism of libido in men and women is complex. Before the menopause, the ovaries produce oestrogen and progesterone. They also produce significant amounts of testosterone; although smaller quantities than in men. Oestrogen and testosterone, together with an enormous number of other physical and psychological variables increase libido. After the menopause, all three hormones are reduced, as is libido in many women. The loss of sexual desire and the feeling of loss of sexual attractiveness to men may have a circular effect on psychological symptoms.

Oestrogen replacement may improve sex drive in many women but a greater proportion will require testosterone. This is not acceptable to many women and so psychological or psychosexual counselling may be more appropriate for such a couple.

When testosterone therapy is needed and acceptable, this is less easy than conventional oestrogen therapy. Presently, testosterone can only be given transdermally. Testosterone implants given with oestradiol are extremely effective and require nothing to be taken regularly, although a 6-monthly minor surgical procedure must be undergone.

Transdermal patches and gels of testosterone have been used less successfully and currently they are licensed only for use in men. This is likely to change. In the meantime, doses need to be adjusted downwards.

In addition to the central endocrine effects of hormones on sex drive, gynaecologists will need to consider the local physical effects of oestrogen deficiency and their effects on sex drive and function.

Oestrogen deficiency can give rise to vaginal thinning, tearing, pain and failure of lubrication before and during intercourse. These physical effects can give rise to secondary psychological effects, further reduction in libido and vaginismus being the most obvious. The vaginal condition can be reversed using systemic oestrogen, although this is not always successful alone and oestradiol pessaries and creams may be required. Additionally, simple preparations such as vaginal lubricants are extremely valuable if the oestrogen effect is insufficient or declined by the woman.

Alternatives to oestrogen preparations and mood disorders

Women may be unhappy to take systemic oestrogen, which has not been shown to have a true antidepressant effect. As we have seen, it is possible that the so-called antidepressant effect of oestrogen is mediated via its effect on the alleviation of vasomotor symptoms and insomnia – there is a continuing debate in this area. It is, however, likely that oestrogen and testosterone have direct antidepressant actions. In women who decline HRT, the question arises whether or not they should be prescribed sedatives, hypnotics or antidepressants. It is thought that these drugs are less effective than oestrogen replacement though the SSRIs such as fluoxetine may benefit depression whilst venlafaxine (a serotonin and noradrenaline reuptake inhibitor) will improve depression and there is also limited evidence that it will improve flushes. Both of these drugs are certainly used frequently and there may be a synergistic or enhancing effect of oestrogen and SSRIs together.

The role of counselling, stress management and psychotherapy should also be considered but, again, research evidence is limited.

There are many unproven nonmedical techniques that have been claimed to be useful for all menopause symptoms. Some of these include homoeopathy, dietary measures and supplements, acupuncture, phyto-estrogens and progesterone creams. Supportive data are awaited for most of these treatments.

References

1. Bäckström T. Symptoms related to the menopause and sex steroid treatments. *Ciba Found Symp* 1995;191:171–86.
2. Stuenkel CA. Menopause and estrogen replacement therapy. *Psychiatr Clin North Am* 1989;12:133–52.
3. World Health Organization. *Research on the Menopause*. Geneva: WHO; 1981.
4. Kaufert PA, Gilbert P, Tate R. The Manitoba project; a re-examination of the link between menopause and depression. *Maturitas* 1992;14:143–55.
5. Avis NE, Brambilla D, McKinlay SM, Vass K. A longitudinal analysis of the association between menopause and depression. Results from the Massachusetts Women's Health Study. *Ann Epidemiol* 1994;4:214–20.
6. Hunter M. The South-east England longitudinal study of the climacteric and postmenopause. *Maturitas* 1992;14:117–26.
7. Holte A. Influences of natural menopause on health complaints; a prospective study of healthy Norwegian women. *Maturitas* 1992;14:127–41.
8. Ballinger CB. Psychiatric aspects of the menopause. *Br J Psychiatry* 1990;156:773–87.
9. Dennerstein L, Smith AM, Morse C, Burger H, Green A, Hopper J, *et al.* Menopausal symptoms in Australian women. *Med J Aust* 1993;159:232–6.
10. McKinlay SM, Brambilla DJ, Posner JG. The normal menopause transition. *Maturitas* 1992;14:103–15.
11. Collins A, Landgren BM. Reproductive health, use of estrogen and experience of symptoms in perimenopausal women: a population-based study. *Maturitas*

1994;20:101–11.
12. Meltzer HY. Role of serotonin in depression. *Ann N Y Acad Sci* 1990;600:486–99.
13. Frackiewicz EJ, Cutler NR. Women's health care during the perimenopause. *J Am Pharm Assoc (Wash)* 2000;40:800–11.
14. Pop VJ, Maartens LH, Leusink G, van Son MJ, Knottnerus AA, Ward AM, *et al.* Are autoimmune thyroid dysfunction and depression related? *J Clin Endocrinol Metab* 1998;83:3194–7.
15. Bachmann G, Bancroft J, Braunstein G, Burger H, Davis S, Dennerstein L, *et al.* Female androgen insufficiency: the Princeton consensus statement on definition, classification, and assessment. *Fertil Steril* 2002;77:660–5.
16. Davis SR, Burger HG. The role of androgen therapy. *Best Pract Res Clin Endocrinol Metab* 2003;17:165–75.
17. Halbreich U, Kahn LS. Role of estrogen in the aetiology and treatment of mood disorders. *CNS Drugs* 2001;15:797–817.
18. Soares CN, Poitras JR, Prouty J. Effect of reproductive hormones and selective estrogen receptor modulators on mood during menopause. *Drugs Aging* 2003;20:85–100.
19. Khastgir G, Studd J. Hysterectomy, ovarian failure, and depression. *Menopause* 1998;5:113–22.
20. Zweifel JE, O'Brien WH. A meta-analysis of the effect of HRT upon depressed mood. *Psychoneuroendocrinology* 1997;22:189–212.
21. Yonkers KA, Bradshaw KD, Halbreich U. Oestrogens, progestins and mood. In: Steiner M, Yonkers K, Eriksson E, editors. *Mood Disorders in Women.* London: Martin Dunitz; 2000. p. 207–32.
22. Westlund TL, Parry BL. Does estrogen enhance the antidepressant effects of fluoxetine? *J Affect Disord* 2003;77:87–92.
23. Morris E, Rymer J. Menopausal symptoms. *Clin Evidence* 2003;9:2074–86.
24. Haskell SG, Richardson ED, Horwitz RI. The effect of ORT on cognitive function in women: a critical review of the literature. *J Clin Epidemiol* 1997;50:1249–64.
25. Polo-Kantola P, Erkkola R, Irjala K, Pullinen S, Virtanen I, Polo O. Effect of short-term transdermal estrogen replacement therapy on sleep: a randomized, double-blind crossover trial in postmenopausal women. *Fertil Steril* 1999;71:873–80.
26. Karlberg J, Mattsson L, Wiklund I. A quality of life perspective on who benefits from estradiol replacement therapy. *Acta Obstet Gynecol Scand* 1995;74:367–72.
27. Derman RJ, Dawood MY, Stone S. Quality of life during sequential hormone replacement therapy: a placebo-controlled study. *Int J Fertil Menopausal Stud* 1995;40:73–8.
28. Hilditch JR, Lewis J, Ross AH, Peter A, van Maris B, Franssen E, *et al.* A comparison of the effects of oral conjugated equine estrogen and transdermal estradiol-17 beta combined with an oral progestin on quality of life in postmenopausal women. *Maturitas* 1996;24:177–84.
29. Wiklund I, Karlberg J, Mattsson L. Quality of life of postmenopausal women on a regimen of transdermal estradiol therapy: a double-blind placebo-controlled study. *Am J Obstet Gynecol* 1993;168:824–30.

9　Substance use disorders

Epidemiology

Specialists in obstetrics and gynaecology should be aware of the nature and extent of substance misuse in the UK. It is important to realise the scale of the problem, especially in young people, including young women of reproductive age. The trend is towards increased use over the last decade. Polydrug misuse (the 'pick and mix' phenomenon) is common.

The age at which young people start substance misuse is decreasing. Young people misuse for many reasons: because their friends do, out of curiosity, to feel good, because of low self-esteem, poor achievement at school, family history of drugs or drink, violence in the family and emotional distress.

The Confidential Enquiries into Maternal Deaths (2000–2002) found that, when all deaths up to 1 year from delivery were taken into account, psychiatric illness was not only the leading cause of indirect death, but also the leading cause of maternal deaths overall. Of the 391 women whose deaths were reported to the Enquiries, 8% were substance misusers.

An overwhelming 20% of 13 year olds and 25% of 15 year olds smoke daily. For the first time girls have overtaken boys in prevalence of cigarette use. Nearly 50% of young men aged 16–24 years drink over the 'safe' recommended limit of 3 units of alcohol per day for adult men. Some 40% of young women drink more than 2 units per day (or the safe limit for adult women). Twenty-four percent (2.3 million) of 16–24 year olds have used an illicit drug in the previous year. Perhaps unsurprisingly therefore, teenagers in the UK have the highest rates of drug and alcohol use in Europe and approximately 50% of teenagers will have a substance problem, particularly alcohol and cigarettes. It has become apparent that the most highly prevalent problem is not illegal drugs but rather legal drugs such as cigarettes and alcohol.

Diagnostic terms

In the term 'substance' we include nicotine, alcohol, amphetamines, cannabis, benzodiazepines, codeine-based over the counter drugs, cocaine and crack cocaine, ecstasy, LSD, heroin and other opiates, methadone, prescribed medications (whether taken compliantly or not) and solvents.

The term 'substance use' indicates that the substance is medically compliant with prescriber's instructions, socially in accordance with cultural norms and legally acceptable, i.e. licit. Therefore, the term 'misuse' indicates that use is medically, legally and socially unacceptable and that evidence points to the potentially harmful nature of the substance if use is continued on a long-term basis.

It is vital to be able to differentiate between misuse and dependence. In general, a diagnosis of 'dependence' (or addiction) indicates the problem is more severe with more associated problems. Hence, treatment options differ. For instance, a definite diagnosis of dependence is required before pharmacological treatments can be prescribed. At least three criteria must be present in the previous year for a diagnosis of 'dependence' to be reached. These are:

- compulsion or a strong desire to take the substance

- difficulties in controlling the use of the substance

- a withdrawal syndrome when substance use has ceased or been reduced; the individual may also report the use of substances to relieve the withdrawal symptoms

- evidence of tolerance such that higher doses are required to achieve the same effect

- neglect of interests and an increased amount of time taken to obtain the substance or recover from its effects.

- persistent substance use despite evidence of its harmful consequences.

The assessment process

The assessment is considered part of the treatment process (Box 9.1). The non-judgemental and non-confrontational style as well as the sensitivity of the interviewer powerfully determines how a patient, who may be ambivalent, reacts to the situation. The key is to engage the patient with the recognition that the assessment and treatment may be continuous and over the long term. Furthermore, if substance misuse is identified early, there is less likelihood of progression to more severe conditions with associated psychological, social and physical problems.

BOX 9.1 ASSESSMENT

Each substance should be discussed separately:

- alcohol
- amphetamines
- benzodiazepines
- cannabis
- cocaine
- 'ecstasy'
- heroin and other opiates
- methadone
- nicotine
- over-the-counter medication
- prescribed medication, including compliance

Each substance should be assessed regarding:

- age of initiation – when 'first tried'
- age of onset of weekend use
- age of onset of weekly use
- age of onset of daily use
- pattern of use during each day
- route of use, e.g. oral, smoking, snorting, intramuscular, intravenous
- age of onset of specific withdrawal symptoms and dependence syndrome features
- current use over previous day, week, month
- current cost of use
- maximum use ever
- how is the substance use being funded?
- periods of abstinence
- triggers to relapse
- preferred substance(s) and reasons

Details of previous treatment episodes for substance misuse:

- dates
- service
- practitioner details
- treatment interventions
- success or otherwise

Substance misuse may produce, reflect or mask a range of social, psychological and physical problems (Table 9.1). Indeed, more often than not, the substance use is not the patient's only, or even most serious, problem. Thus, identification of the underlying or associated problems is just as important in the treatment plan. Management must be based on a balanced systematic assessment of clinical history, examination and biochemical results. Symptoms of intoxication and withdrawal of the different substances are listed in Table 9.2.

Table 9.1. Social, psychological and physical problems associated with substance misuse

Type of problem	Manifestation
Social	Parental conflict, separation, divorce, physical or sexual abuse, neglect, unemployment, truancy, criminal involvement, prostitution and crime to fund habit, poor monitoring or supervision of children by parents
Psychological	Psychological distress, symptoms of psychiatric disorder, or even suicide or self-harming behaviour. Substances may produce psychological symptoms as a result of intoxication, withdrawal and dependence symptoms
Physical	Physical damage results from infection, under the skin or vascular injection, smoking or inhalation. Venous damage with difficult venous access for blood sampling and intravenous drugs, blood and fluids

Substance misuse in pregnancy

ALCOHOL MISUSE

Antenatal alcohol use is the leading preventable cause of birth defects, mental restriction and neurodevelopmental disorders. Yet half of pregnant women report drinking during pregnancy, one-fifth of these drink at moderate or high levels and one-fifth report continued drinking into pregnancy.[2,3] In the USA, the incidence of children affected by prenatal alcohol exposure ranges from 0.5–3.0 births per 1000, although the overall rate in the Western world has been estimated at 0.33 per 1000 live births.[4] In addition to the full syndrome, there are three to five children per 1000 who will exhibit less severe effects termed alcohol-related birth defects. Authors have described the dysmorphic features, growth restriction and CNS problems associated with fetal alcohol syndrome.[5,6] Dysmorphic features include microcephaly, micro-ophthalmia, thin upper lip and a flattening of the

Table 9.2. Symptoms of intoxication and withdrawal of different substances

Substance	Intoxication	Withdrawal
Alcohol	Disinhibition, argumentativeness, aggression, interference with personal functioning, lability of mood, impaired judgment and attention, unsteady gait and difficulty in standing, slurred speech, nystagmus, decreased level of consciousness, flushed face, conjunctival injection	Tremor: tongue, eyelids, hands Agitation, insomnia, malaise Convulsions Visual, auditory, tactile illusions or hallucinations
Opiates	Apathy, sedation, disinhibition, psychomotor retardation, impaired attention, impaired judgment, interference with personal functioning, drowsiness, slurred speech, papillary constriction, decreased level of consciousness	Craving, sneezing, yawning, runny eyes, muscle aches, abdominal pains, nausea, vomiting, diarrhoea, pupillary dilatation, goose flesh, recurrent chills, restless sleep
Cannabis	Euphoria and disinhibition, anxiety and agitation, suspiciousness and paranoid ideation, impaired reaction time, judgment and attention, hallucinations with preserved orientation, depersonalisation and derealisation, increased appetite, dry mouth, conjunctival injection and tachycardia	Anxiety, irritability, tremor, sweating, muscle aches
Nicotine	Insomnia, bizarre dreams, fluctuating mood, derealisation, interference with personal functioning, nausea, sweating, tachycardia and cardiac arrythmias	Craving, malaise or weakness, anxiety, irritability, moodiness, insomnia, increased appetite, increased cough and mouth ulceration, difficulty in concentrating
Stimulants	Euphoria and increased energy, hypervigilance, repetitive stereotyped behaviours, grandiose beliefs and actions, paranoid ideation, abusiveness, aggression and argumentativeness, auditory, tactile and visual hallucinations, sweats, chills, muscular weakness, nausea or vomiting, weight loss, pupillary dilatation, convulsions, tachycardia, arrythmias, chest pain, hypertension, agitation	Lethargy, psychomotor retardation or agitation, craving, increased appetite, insomnia or hypersomnia, bizarre and unpleasant dreams

midface. CNS effects include mental restriction, hyperactivity and attention deficits, poor impulse control, and language and motor development delays.[7] Affected children continue to manifest developmental disabilities, psychiatric disorders and cognitive delay as they mature. In terms of dysmorphic features, those who are more severely damaged also show the more prevalent and marked psychiatric symptoms. Milder difficulties in mothers drinking more than 250 grams of alcohol per week have been noted, such as poor attention span, distractibility and poorer performance on IQ and neurobehavioural tests. Streissguth *et al.*, in a 14-year follow-up study, identified dose response effects of alcohol prenatally on neurobehavioural attention, speed of information processing and learning function at 14 years.[8,9]

The most effective way of detecting heavy alcohol consumption is the TACE (tolerance, annoyed, cut down, eye opener) questionnaire, which can be used to screen either the whole population or targeted at those women with growth-impaired fetuses. Only four questions are required, as shown in Box 9.2. A total score of greater than or equal to two points is considered positive and correctly identifies over 70% of heavy drinkers during pregnancy.

BOX 9.2. TACE

T How many drinks does it take to make you feel high (**tolerance**)?

A Have people **annoyed** you by criticising your drinking?

C Have you ever felt you ought to **cut down** on your drinking?

E Have you ever had a drink first thing in the morning to steady your nerves or get rid of a hangover (**eye opener**)?

There is no conclusive evidence of adverse effects in either growth or IQ at levels of consumption below 120 g (15 units) per week. Nonetheless, it is recommended that women should be careful about alcohol consumption in pregnancy and limit this to no more than one standard drink per day.[10]

NICOTINE MISUSE

Exposure to nicotine during pregnancy results in low birth weight and intrauterine growth restriction associated with developmental delay. A recurring theme is the association between maternal smoking during pregnancy and sudden infant death syndrome,[11] and the correlation of passive smoking with respiratory difficulties in infants. Duration of smoking, exposure to environmental smoke (such as smoking in partners and family), self-efficacy and educational methods have been demonstrated to influence the mother's reduction in nicotine use during and after pregnancy.[12]

ILLEGAL SUBSTANCE MISUSE

A classic opiate abstinence withdrawal syndrome occurs in at least 50% of babies born to mothers using opiates. No clear teratogenic effect has been identified, although consistent findings include low birth weight, prematurity and reduced intrauterine growth.[11] Cannabis exposure is related to shorter gestation and low birth weight and later effects on the central nervous system, cognitive development and behaviour.[13–15] A mild withdrawal syndrome has been reported and disturbed sleep with potentiation of the effects of alcohol on the fetus have been described.[16,17] Although 'crack babies' have attracted attention in the popular press, no consistent constellation of findings in the developmental outcome of those prenatally exposed to cocaine has emerged when compared with matched controls. Maternal cocaine use is associated with restricted intrauterine brain growth[11,18] and placental abruption.[19] However, cognitive effects may be related to associated environmental risk, social status and exposure to multiple and cumulative risks, which compromise outcomes and which may overshadow any prenatal effect from cocaine.[20] It should also be noted that 'ecstasy' is associated with congenital cardiovascular and musculoskeletal abnormalities.[21] Thus, prenatal exposure should be seen as a possible marker for multiple medical and social risk factors, for example, social isolation, maternal psychopathology, violence and child abuse.

Treatment

WHEN PHARMACOLOGICAL INTERVENTIONS ARE REQUIRED

As described above, a diagnosis of dependence will suggest the need to use pharmacological agents for a variety of indications. The appropriateness of particular pharmacological interventions and the need for supervision by a carer (depending on the age, competence and stage of pregnancy of the woman) require careful consideration. Medication should be carefully monitored, with regular review of urine and blood tests. Irregular chaotic drug use is not an indication for substitute medication.

REASONS WHY INTERVENTIONS ARE NOT OFFERED AND SOUGHT

Pregnancy offers a window of opportunity for the treatment of substance problems because pharmacological, behavioural and social interventions can routinely be offered during pregnancy. If this does not take place, it may partly be related to inadequacy of screening, in depth assessment and care planning, and to the absence of coordinated services. However, it may also be related to parental concerns about the health of the baby, sensitivities about parenting ability, and inability to access proper care.

COORDINATION OF THE CARE PACKAGE

If a young pregnant user presents to services, the principle is synchronisation of the care package. It is helpful to have local protocols in place that routinely involve practitioners from obstetric, substance misuse and primary care services, such as the community midwife, health visitor, general practitioner, and from paediatric, psychiatric and social services if required. Limiting the number of hospital visits by synchronising and streamlining appointments reduces non-attendance.

BASIC ISSUES AROUND PREGNANCY

The substance misuse, psychiatric, obstetric and medical assessments are basic issues to be addressed. Treatment during pregnancy, labour and after delivery should be discussed, carefully planned and harmonised if there is time. Young pregnant users do present late in pregnancy or occasionally at delivery. Aspects relating to labour such as drug and alcohol withdrawal (especially if there are obstetric emergencies), the need for arrangements for substitute prescribing, the type of analgesia, the mother's viral status and views about delivery are some issues that need to be addressed. Thereafter, breastfeeding, probable adjustment of medication, immunisation, contraception and arrangements for discharge and follow-up need review, particularly if the baby has been in the special care baby unit and there are child protection issues.

CONTROLLED TRIALS IN PREGNANCY

As well as the need to evaluate treatment interventions in young people, there is the necessity to pay particular attention to the special needs of pregnant young people, although of course not all users are young. There is a paucity of well-controlled trials.

The first randomised trial comparing brief intervention and comprehensive assessment with assessment only for drinking found reductions in both groups antenatally. However, women who were abstinent prior to assessment, and who received a brief intervention, maintained higher rates of abstinence in the pregnancy than the control group.[22] Administration of brief interventions to reduce or stop alcohol use is advisable. Occasionally, detoxification is necessary.

Randomised controlled trials of nicotine replacement therapy in this group are required. Given the adverse consequences, it is sensible to consider the use of nicotine replacement if there is no response to behavioural interventions.[23] Indeed, National Institute for Clinical Excellence (NICE) guidance (2002) has recommended that those under 18 years and pregnant and breastfeeding women may be prescribed nicotine replacement therapy on the recommendation of a medical practitioner.[24] Even if nicotine replacement therapy has no eventual impact on cigarette addiction, substitute therapy may be shown to improve obstetric, neonatal and developmental outcome.

Methadone treatment as part of a comprehensive package of care has been shown to improve birth outcomes and maternal psychosocial function.[25] There are problems related to the development of a prolonged neonatal withdrawal syndrome, which occurs in more than 60% of infants and which may lengthen hospitalisation. For this reason, buprenorphine has been explored and found to be safe and effective in the mother, fetus and infant during conception, throughout pregnancy and in the early neonatal period. Although it is still not certain how methadone and buprenorphine compare in terms of outcome measures, buprenorphine has a further advantage that in the UK it is licensed for use in the 16–18 years age group.[26–28]

Psychosocial interventions

Psychosocial interventions remain more important because, once detoxification, reduction or maintenance is established, sustained improvement depends upon behavioural change. Although most practitioners are concerned about the 'prescribing' aspects, understandably, because of safety issues, in fact, the majority of treatment interventions are 'psychological'.

BRIEF INTERVENTIONS

Most generalist obstetricians and their teams can offer 5–10 minutes of brief advice or information regarding the substance problem. This may include the provision of information about the risks to the fetus and personal risks of substances, information about 'safe' levels of drinking, provision of self-help materials on ways to stop smoking, or on safer injecting practices. The practitioner may, in addition, offer the opportunity for the patient to express anxieties or discuss the results of screening or blood tests.

ABSTINENCE OR HARM-REDUCTION GOALS

Assessment of degree of 'motivation to change', although often tricky to establish, can point to the next step. Women should be encouraged to decide whether abstinence or reduction is their 'goal'. If harm reduction or minimisation is the priority, information about immunisation, vaccination and contraception is important.

ABSTINENCE AS THE GOAL

If abstinence is the 'goal' and no pharmacological treatment is required, a 'quit' date should be set. Patients should get rid of and avoid alcohol, cigarettes or drugs, and work on alternative strategies for coping. These would include keeping a diary about how much they are using, setting limits for use, controlling rate of intake, learning refusal skills, assertiveness and relaxation training, anger management, alternative coping skills with new or different rewards and identifying and challenging negative automatic thoughts which predispose to substance misuse.

Specialist treatment interventions and settings

Specialist treatment interventions may include both intensive psychological and pharmacological interventions. In certain circumstances, the woman has to be admitted to a specialist inpatient unit. This is usually in the case of severe dependence on one or more substances, severe physical illness, comorbid psychiatric illness, abuse of multiple substances, frequent relapsing substance misuse and unstable social circumstances.

If more intensive psychological support, either individual, group or family work is required, this will be assessed and organised by the specialist service during an admission, on an outpatient basis or in the community. If the nature and extent of substance problems are such that specialist input is required, assistance in arranging this, as well as continued support and encouragement, should be offered.

TREATMENT DOES WORK, AND AN OPTIMISTIC APPROACH IS WARRANTED

That 'treatment works' should be emphasised, especially if the woman has had previous negative experiences. This may be especially pertinent at particular times, such as pregnancy, or in relation to particular behaviours and lifestyle issues like prostitution and sex working. It may be necessary to arrange the first appropriate consultation with the specialist service and to accompany the woman.

A model of a pregnant drug users' service

At the North Staffordshire Hospitals, the pregnant drug users' service is provided by a specialist substance misuse unit and a specialised antenatal clinic. These units are in close proximity on the hospital site so that pregnant women can be seen in both units within an hour. The multidisciplinary team that manages this service includes a consultant addiction psychiatrist, an associate specialist in substance misuse, a family therapist, a consultant obstetrician and a named midwife based at the maternity unit. The service has close links with the neonatology unit. The objective of the service is to target the social, physical, psychological and pharmacological needs of the mother, fetus, neonate and family.

Women treated at the pregnant drug users' service are reviewed weekly in the substance misuse unit. The centre offers a range of physical, psychosocial and pharmacological interventions on an in- or outpatient basis. Opiate-dependent patients are offered substitution therapy with either methadone or buprenorphine. Pharmacological treatments for smoking cessation and alcohol dependence are also provided by the centre. Women are reviewed in the antenatal clinic every 2 weeks, starting from 24 weeks of gestation, with serial ultrasound scans to monitor fetal growth and liquor volume and more detailed assessment with biophysical profiles, cardiotocogram (CTG) and Doppler assessments where the scan identifies a problem. Review by both units is organised to take place on the same day to decrease the risk of defaulting antenatal appointments. Methadone or buprenorphine prescriptions for women at high risk of defaulting are given after the antenatal appointment has been completed.

Provided that fetal growth is appropriate and there are no obstetric or social indications for induction of labour, we would aim for spontaneous onset of labour and vaginal delivery. The fetus is continuously monitored in labour and pethidine pain relief is avoided. A neonatologist reviews and assesses babies over the following few days for any signs or symptoms of neonatal abstinence syndrome.

Summary

Until systematic controlled studies are undertaken, clinical decisions have to be made based on whether the potential benefits from pharmacological treatments outweigh the risks associated with continued substance misuse during pregnancy. Psychosocial interventions remain the mainstay but risk management is particularly important if substance misuse is chaotic or dependent, and pharmacological agents are being prescribed.

References

1. Lewis G, editor. *Why Mothers Die 2000–2002. The Sixth Report of the Confidential Enquiries into Maternal Deaths in the United Kingdom*. London: RCOG Press; 2004.
2. Floyd RL, Decoufle P, Hungerford DW. Alcohol use prior to pregnancy recognition. *Am J Prev Med* 1999;17:101–7.
3. Morse BA, Hutchins E. Reducing complications from alcohol use through screening. *J Am Med Women's Assoc* 2000;55:225–7.
4. Abel EL, Sokol R. A revised conservative estimate of the incidence of fetal alcohol syndrome and its economic impact. *Alcohol Clin Exp Res* 1991;15:514–24.
5. Jones K, Smith D. Recognition of the fetal alcohol syndrome in early infancy. *Lancet* 1973;ii:999–1001.
6. Lemoine P, Harousseau H, Borteyru JP, Menuet JC. Children of alcoholic parents-observed anomalies: discussion of 127 cases. *Ther Drug Monit* 2003;25:132–6.
7. Young NK. Effects of alcohol and other drugs on children. *J Psychoactive Drugs* 1997;29:23–42.
8. Streissguth AP, Barr HM, Sampson PD, Bookstein FL. Prenatal alcohol and offspring development: the first fourteen years. *Drug Alcohol Depend* 1994;36:89–99.
9. Streissguth AP, Sampson PD, Olson HC, Bookstein FL, Barr HM, Scott M, *et al.* Maternal drinking during pregnancy: attention and short-term memory in 14-year-old offspring: a longitudinal prospective study. *Alcohol Clin Exp Res* 1994;18:202–18.
10. Royal College of Obstetricians and Gynaecologists. *Alcohol Consumption in Pregnancy*. Guideline No. 9. London: RCOG; 1999.
11. Bauer C. Perinatal effects of prenatal drug exposure. *Clin Perinatol* 1999;26:87–106.
12. Woodby LL, Windsor RA, Snyder SW, Kohler CL, Diclemente CC. Predictors of smoking cessation during pregnancy. *Addiction* 1999;94:283–92.
13. Fergusson DM, Horwood LJ, Northstone K, the ALSPAC study team. Maternal use of cannabis and pregnancy outcome. *BJOG* 2002;109:21–7.
14. Martin BR, Hall W. The health effects of cannabis: key issues of policy relevance. *United Nations Office on Drugs and Crime Bulletin on Narcotics* 1997;(1) [www.unodc.org/unodc/en/bulletin/bulletin_1997-01-01_1_page005.html].
15. Scher MS, Richardson GA, Coble PA, Day NL, Stoffer DS. The effects of prenatal alcohol and marijuana exposure: disturbances in neonatal sleep cycling and arousal. *Pediatr Res* 1988;24:101–5.
16. Fried PA. Marijuana use during pregnancy: consequences for the offspring. *Semin Perinatol* 1991;15:280–7.
17. Dahl RE, Scher MS, Williamson D. A longitudinal study of prenatal marijuana use: Effects on sleep and arousal at age 3 years. *Arch Pediatr Med* 1995;149:145–50.
18. Bateman DA, Chriboga CA. Dose response effect of cocaine on newborn head circumference. *Pediatrics* 2000;106:33–9.
19. Hladky K, Yankowitz J, Hansen WF. Placental abruption. *Obstet Gynecol Surv* 2002;57:299–305.
20. Tronick E, Beeghly M. Prenatal cocaine exposure, child development, and the

compromising effects of cumulative risk. *Clin Perinatol* 1999;26:151–71.
21. McElhatton PR, Bateman DN, Evans C, Pughe KR, Thomas SH. Congenital anomalies after prenatal ecstasy exposure. *Lancet* 1999;354:1441–2.
22. Chang G, Wilkins-Haug L, Berman S, Goetz MA. Brief intervention for alcohol use in pregnancy: A randomised trial. *Addiction* 1999;94:1499–508.
23. Wisborg K, Henriksen TB, Jespersen LB, Secher NJ. Nicotine patches for pregnant smokers: a randomized controlled study. *Obstet Gynecol* 2000;96:967–71.
24. National Institute for Clinical Excellence. *Nicotine Replacement Therapy (NRT) and Bupropion for Smoking Cessation*. Technology Appraisal Guidance No. 39. London: NICE; 2002 [www.nice.org.uk/page.aspx?o=30590].
25. Batey RG, Weissel K. A 40 month follow up of pregnant drug using women treated at Westmead Hospital. *Drug Alcohol Rev* 1993;12:265–70.
26. Fischer G, Johnson RE, Eder H, Jagsch R, Peternell A, Weninger M, *et al.* Treatment of opioid dependent pregnant women with buprenorphine. *Addiction* 2000;95:239–44.
27. Schindler SD, Eder H, Ortner R. Neonatal outcome following buprenorphine maintenance during conception and throughout pregnancy. *Addiction* 2003;98:103–10.
28. Fischer G. Treatment of opioid dependence in pregnant women. *Addiction* 2000;95:1141–44.

10 Other disorders

Sexual dysfunction

According to the WHO International Classification of Diseases, 10th edition,[1] the following criteria are required for the diagnosis of sexual dysfunction:

- The individual cannot participate in a relationship as he or she would like.
- The sexual dysfunction is frequently present but may be absent on some occasions.
- The dysfunction has been present for at least 6 months.
- The dysfunction cannot be accounted for entirely by a physical disorder, drug treatment or any other mental or behavioural disorder.

TYPES OF SEXUAL DYSFUNCTIONS

Lack or loss of sexual desire

In addition to the general criteria of sexual dysfunction, this disorder is characterised by a low urge to engage in sexual activity. The lack of desire makes initiation of sexual interaction less likely. Loss of desire may be with a particular partner or total. In cases of a total loss of sexual desire, a thorough medical history and examination is essential to rule out physical causes such as chronic pain, hormonal disturbances or effects of drugs. Psychiatric assessment is important to exclude a depressive episode.

It is important to determine the individual's motivation to seek treatment. Quite often an individual will seek treatment because of pressure from his or her partner. If the individual does not have motivation to deal with the problem, the prognosis is likely to be less favourable.

Sexual aversion

Sexual aversion is fear and anxiety about sexual interaction with a partner to the extent that sexual activity is avoided. In addition to this, the general criteria of sexual dysfunction should be met before the diagnosis is made.

Lack of sexual enjoyment

The general criteria for sexual dysfunction must be met. In addition, the genital response (orgasm and/or ejaculation) occurs during sexual stimulation but is not accompanied by pleasurable sensations or feelings of pleasant excitement.

Failure of genital response

Among women, the main dysfunction is vaginal dryness. This problem can be secondary to anxiety or exacerbated by pathological factors such as infection and oestrogen deficiency. The main dysfunction in men is erectile failure (inability to develop or maintain an erection). Erectile failure may be primary (the man has never been able to sustain an erection) or secondary. In addition, the dysfunction may be total or situational (the man is only unable to sustain an erection in certain circumstances). Primary total erectile failure is rare and usually has a physical basis. Situational dysfunction is likely to have a psychological cause.

Orgasmic dysfunction

In orgasmic dysfunction there is either absence or marked delay of orgasm, which takes one of the following forms:

- orgasm has never been experienced in any situation
- orgasmic dysfunction has developed after a period of relatively normal response:
  ○ general – orgasmic dysfunction occurs in all situations and with any partner
  ○ situational – orgasm does not happen in certain situations.

Orgasmic dysfunction in men is also referred to as inhibited ejaculation and is thought to be a relatively rare dysfunction. However, in women it is one of the most common sexual complaints.

Premature ejaculation

Premature ejaculation is commonly described as the inability to control ejaculation adequately for both partners to enjoy sexual interaction. In some cases ejaculation may occur before or immediately after penetration or may even occur in the absence of an erection. Ejaculation may appear to be premature if prolonged stimulation is required for development of an erection but, in this case, the primary problem is delayed erection rather than premature ejaculation. Rapid ejaculation is common in young men during their first sexual encounters and most men will subsequently gain control over the speed of ejaculation.

Premature ejaculation is usually a primary problem and is unlikely that it has an organic basis. This dysfunction can occur as a secondary problem during a time of stress or can occur transiently when a man's frequency of sexual activity is reduced.

Non-organic vaginismus

In addition to the general criteria of sexual dysfunction, there is spasm of the perivaginal muscles, sufficient to prevent penile entry or to make it uncomfortable. The dysfunction takes one of the following forms:

- normal response has never been experienced

- vaginismus has developed after a period of relatively normal response:
  - when vaginal entry is not attempted, a normal sexual response may occur
  - any attempt at sexual contact leads to generalized fear and efforts to avoid vaginal entry (e.g., spasm of the adductor muscles of the thighs).

Events or thoughts that may be associated with vaginismus include:

- fear of sex instilled by family and friends that the first intercourse will be painful and bloody

- previous rape or attempt of rape

- the belief that premarital sex is sinful is so ingrained that even when intercourse is sanctioned by marriage it is difficult to relax physically and mentally

- fear of pregnancy and normal labour

- childhood punishment for masturbation.

Physical examination is important to exclude an organic cause for the problem.

Non-organic dyspareunia

Pain is experienced at the entry of the vagina, either throughout sexual intercourse or only when deep thrusting of the penis occurs. This pain should not be secondary to vaginismus or failure of lubrication. Gynaecological examination and investigations might be needed to exclude organic causes of dyspareunia.

TREATMENT

The general gynaecologist is unlikely to posses the skills necessary to assess and treat the complex problems associated with sexual dysfunction. However, they will be able to exclude organic and/or physical problems that might be the underlying cause of sexual dysfunction. The general gynaecologist will also be able to determine the individual's motivation to seek treatment, provide information about phases of sexual function and, most importantly, arrange referral for expert treatment.

Psycho-oncology

EFFECT OF STRESS AND DEPRESSION ON CANCER DEVELOPMENT AND PROGRESSION

Studies linking stress and immune-related illnesses in humans are difficult to interpret because of the existence of a variety of confounding factors that are difficult to control for. Prospective studies in humans on the development of cancer are mixed. Some studies have indicated a relation between depressive symptoms (presumably secondary to increased stress and inability to cope) and cancer development; others have been unable to replicate these findings.[2-4]

The links between psychological features and risk of cancer development and progression have been studied through psycho-neuroimmunology. It is hypothesised that the persistent activation of the hypothalamic-pituitary-adrenal (HPA) axis in the chronic stress response and in depression probably impairs the immune response and contributes to the development and progression of some types of cancer.[5]

Studies in human cancer have linked psychological factors and outcome by the effect of the former on the immune system. Spiegel *et al.*[6] tested a structured group intervention in patients with metastatic breast cancer. The group who received the intervention had approximately double the survival time. Other studies have linked psychological interventions in cancer patients with enhanced T-cell function, mixed lymphocyte responsiveness and greater natural killer cell activity.[7-8]

Hence, stress and depression may affect the process of immune surveillance or the mechanisms that deal with somatic mutations and genomic instability by decreasing cytotoxic T-cell and natural-killer-cell activities.[5]

PSYCHOLOGICAL IMPACT OF CANCER AND ITS TREATMENT

The diagnosis of cancer has major implications for individuals, their families and friends. Although individuals are in a crisis they are required to adapt quickly to catastrophic news. They must try to control the level of emotional distress while making crucial treatment decisions. Major concerns are fear of death, dependency, disfigurement, disability and abandonment, as well as disruptions in relationships, role function and financial status. Moreover, radiotherapy and chemotherapy with the associated adverse effects adds to the negative emotional impact. Even cancer survivors who are cured of cancer may continue to suffer with the psychological impact of their traumatising experience. It is, therefore, essential that a multidisciplinary oncology service has the facilities to offer psychological support to patients and their families.

Psychological disorders in the elderly

With increasing life expectancy secondary to global improvement in health and social conditions, the number of elderly people in the population is increasing. The elderly have a higher incidence of depression, anxiety and cognitive impairment. This is probably secondary to altered cerebral metabolism of monoamines particularly dopamine, serotonin and noradrenaline.[9] These psychological morbidities can impact on how elderly patients present, as well as their management. Depressed patients can present with somatic symptoms, either secondary to somatisation of the disorder or as an exaggeration of the symptoms of a co-existent physical disorder.[10] More seriously, cognitive impairment in the elderly could lead to delay in their management because of a late presentation or a false impression of somatisation by their families or even their health carers.

References

1. World Health Organization. The International Statistical Classification of Diseases and Related Health Problems. 10th ed. Geneva: WHO; 1993 [www.who.int/classifications/icd/en/].

2. Montazeri A, Jarvandi S, Ebrahimi M, Haghighat S, Ansari M. The role of depression in the development of breast cancer: analysis of registry data from a single institute. *Asian Pac J Cancer Prev* 2004;5:316–19.
3. Palapattu GS, Bastian PJ, Slavney PR, Haisfield-Wolfe ME, Walker JM, Brintzenhofeszoc K, *et al.* Preoperative somatic symptoms are associated with disease progression in patients with bladder carcinoma after cystectomy. *Cancer* 2004;101:2209–13.
4. Kruk J, Aboul-Enein HY. Psychological stress and the risk of breast cancer: a case–control study. *Cancer Detect Prev* 2004;28:399–408.
5. Reiche EM, Nunes SO, Morimoto HK. Stress, depression, the immune system, and cancer. *Lancet Oncol* 2004;5:617–25.
6. Spiegel D, Bloom JR, Kraemer HC, Gottheil E. Effect of psychosocial treatment on survival of patients with metastatic breast cancer. *Lancet* 1989;2:888–91.
7. Gruber BL, Hersh SP, Hall NR, Waletzky LR, Kunz JF, Carpenter JK, Kverno KS, Weiss SM. Immunological responses of breast cancer patients to behavioral interventions. *Biofeedback Self Regul* 1993;18:1–22.
8. Fawzy FI, Fawzy NW, Hyun CS, Elashoff R, Guthrie D, Fahey JL, *et al.* Malignant melanoma. Effects of an early structured psychiatric intervention, coping, and affective state on recurrence and survival 6 years later. *Arch Gen Psychiatry* 1993;50:681–9.
9. Gottfries CG. Neurochemical aspects of aging and diseases with cognitive impairment. *J Neurosci Res* 1990;27:541–7.
10. Tebbs VM, Martin AJ. Affective disorders in the elderly: 1000-patient GP trial on a new drug. *Geriatr Med* 1987;17:17–21.

Further reading

Andrews G, Jenkins R, editors. *Management of Mental Disorders*. Sydney and London: World Health Organization Collaborating Centres for Mental Health; 1999.

Brockington I. *Motherhood and Mental Illness*. Oxford: Oxford University Press; 1996.

Cox J, Holden J. *Perinatal Mental Health: A Guide to the Edinburgh Postnatal Depression Scale*. London: Royal College of Psychiatrists; 2003.

Kohen D. Psychotropic medications in pregnancy. *Advances in Psychiatric Treatment* 2004;10:59–66.

Raphael-Leff J. *Psychological Processes of Childbearing*. London: Chapman and Hall; 1991.

Royal College of Psychiatrists. *Perinatal Mental Health Services: Recommendations for Provision of Services for Childbearing Women* . Council Report CR88. April 2001 [www.rcpsych.ac.uk/publications/cr/cr88.htm].

Royal College of Psychologists. *Patients as Parents*. Council Report CR105. June 2002 [www.rcpsych.ac.uk/publications/cr/cr105.htm].

Scottish Intercollegiate Network. *Postnatal Depression and Puerperal Psychosis: A National Clinical Guideline*. SIGN Publication No. 60. Edinburgh: SIGN; 2002 [www.sign.ac.uk/guidelines/fulltext/60/index.html].

Yonkers K, Little B, editors. *Management of Psychiatric Disorders in Pregnancy*. London: Arnold; 2001.

National organisations and support groups

Note: all websites live at time of printing.

EATA (European Association for the Treatment of Addiction UK)
Waterbridge House, 32–36 Loman Street, London SE1 0EE
Telephone: 020 7922 8753
Website: www.eata.org.uk
Helps to ensure that people with substance dependencies get the
treatment they need.

Talk To Frank
Telephone: 0800 776600
Website: talktofrank.com
National helpline providing information on drug-related matters.
Drugs awareness campaign, launched at the end of May 2003. Aimed
at young people and parents who need help. Although the campaign
itself is focused on those who need help with class A drugs: crack
cocaine, heroin and ecstasy, it is there to help all young people who
are having problems with any drugs or with alcohol.

Action on Addiction
Website: www.aona.co.uk
Independent UK research charity dedicated to seeking new ways to
prevent and treat nicotine, alcohol and drug abuse.

Addaction
Website: www.addaction.org.uk
UK charity working solely in the field of drug and alcohol treatment.

Addiction Today
Website: www.addictiontoday.org/modules/AMS
Journal in the UK drugs and alcohol treatment field. Published
bimonthly by the Addiction Recovery Foundation charity, it is
devoted to leading-edge and evidence-based treatment and good

practice. Articles include therapeutic techniques, research, news, diary, complementary medicines, relevant legislation, lists of self-help groups and treatment centres, details of training for professionals and workshops for people in recovery.

Adfam
Telephone: 020 7928 8898
Website: www.adfam.org.uk
National charity working with families affected by drugs and alcohol and a leading agency in substance-related family work. Provides a range of publications and resources for families about substances and criminal justice and operates an online message board and database of local support groups that helps families hear about and talk to people who understand their situation. Also runs direct support services at London prisons for families of prisoners with drug problems that need to talk about prison and drugs.

ALCOWEB
Website: www.alcoweb.com
Portal on alcohol and alcoholism, (English and French versions).

Al-Anon
61 Great Dover Street, London SE1 4YF.
Telephone: 020 7403 0888
Website: www.al-anonuk.org.uk
Offers understanding and support for families and friends of problem drinkers, whether the alcoholic is still drinking or not. Alateen, a part of Al-Anon, is for young people aged 12–20 years who have been affected by someone else's drinking, usually that of a parent.

Alcohol Concern
Waterbridge House, 32–36 Loman Street, London, SE1 0EE.
Telephone: 020 7928 7377
Email: contact@alcoholconcern.org.uk
Website: www.alcoholconcern.org.uk
UK national agency concerned with alcohol misuse and alcohol-related matters. Provides information and encourages debate on the wide range of public policy issues affected by alcohol, including public health, housing, children and families, crime and licensing. Supports specialist and nonspecialist service providers helping to tackle alcohol problems at a local level, while also working to influence national alcohol policy.

Alcohol Focus Scotland
Website: www.alcohol-focus-scotland.org.uk
National body in Scotland dealing with all aspects of alcohol-related problems.

Alcoholics Anonymous
National helpline: 0845 76 97 555
Website: www.alcoholics-anonymous.org.uk (portall); www.aa-uk.org.uk
Self-help organisation for people dependent on alcohol.

British Menopause Society
4–6 Eton Place, Marlow, Buckinghamshire UK SL7 2QA
Telephone: 01628 890199
Website: www.the-bms.org
The BMS is a registered charity dedicated to increasing awareness of postmenopausal healthcare issues, promoting optimal management through conferences, roadshow and publications.

Centre for Drug Research
Website: www.gla.ac.uk/centres/drugmisuse
University of Glasgow research department. Conducts research on the problem of drug misuse within Scotland.

Centre for Research on Drugs and Health Behaviour
Website: www1.imperial.ac.uk/medicine/about/divisions/ephpc/pcsm/research/crdhb/default.html
London-based centre researching into substance use and related social behaviours. Works with drug, alcohol and sexual health agencies and undertakes multi-site, multi-method research studies within the UK and internationally.

Department of Addictive Behaviour (St Georges Hospital Medical School)
Website: www.sgul.ac.uk/depts/addictive-behaviour/frames.htm
Conducts research and training in the field of addictions.

Drinkline
National helpline providing information on alcohol-related issues
Telephone: 0800 917 8282 (9.00am – 11.00pm, Monday to Friday)
Website: www.drinkanddrugs.net
Web portal for substance misuse practitioners, covering the latest
news, training information, research and guidance, jobs vacancies and
more.
Offers the following services: information and self-help materials;
help to callers worried about their own drinking; support to the
family and friends of people who are drinking; advice to callers on
where to go for help. Drinkline is confidential and no names need be
given. Callers to the above number have the option of listening to
recorded information about alcohol or talking to an adviser.

Drug Action Teams
Website: www.addaction.org.uk/Services_DAT.htm
Work locally to deliver the UK drug strategy. The Drug Action Teams
listed represent the areas in which Addaction is already providing
services.

Drug Misuse Information
Website: www.dh.gov.uk/PolicyAndGuidance/
HealthAndSocialCareTopics/SubstanceMisuse/fs/en
Department of Health website for practitioners working in drug
prevention and treatment services.

Drug Misuse Information Scotland
Website: www.drugmisuse.isdscotland.org/smrt/smrt.htm

www.drugs.gov.uk
Provides drugs professionals with the latest news and guidance
from Government about the Drugs Strategy.

Drugs in Britain
Website: www.guardian.co.uk/drugs/0,2759,178206,00.html
Guardian Unlimited Special Report. Online documentary.

DrugScope
Website: www.drugscope.org.uk
UK national agency concerned with drug use and related matters.
Provides quality drug information, promotes effective responses to
drug taking, undertakes research at local, national and international
levels, advises on policy making, encourages informed debate.

**European Working Group on Drugs-Oriented Research
(EWODOR)**
Website: www.dass.stir.ac.uk/DRUGS/Ewodor.htm
Forum for researchers in the field of drug use and related issues.

European Monitoring Centre for Drugs and Drug Abuse
Website: www.emcdda.eu.int
Monitoring drug use and drug-related problems throughout Europe.

ERIT
Website: www.erit.org
Federation of European Professional Associations Working in the
Field of Drug Abuse.

Families Anonymous
Website: www.famanon.org.uk
Helpline: 0845 1200 660
Faxline: +44 (020 7498 1990
Email: office@famanon.org.uk
Self-help organisation for families and friends of people with drug
problems.

Federation of Drug and Alcohol Professionals
Unit 84, 95 Wilton Road, London SW1V 1BZ.
Telephone: 0870 763 6139
Website: www.fdap.org.uk
Email: office@fdap.org.uk
FDAP is the professional body for practitioners in the substance use
field. It is a membership organisation open to practitioners
throughout the field and works to help improve standards of practice
in dealing with people with drug and alcohol problems.

Institute of Alcohol Studies

Alliance House, 12 Caxton Street, London SW1H 0QS.
Telephone: +44 (0) 207 222 4001
Email: info@ias.org.uk
Website: www.ias.org.uk
Educational body with the basic aims of increasing knowledge of alcohol and the social and health consequences of its misuse and encouraging and supporting the adoption of effective measures for the management and prevention of alcohol-related problems.

London Drug And Alcohol Network

Website: www.ldan.org.uk
Provides advice, information and support to those working directly with people who have drug and alcohol problems in London.

Mainliners

95 New Kent Road, London SE1 4AG.
Telephone: +44 (0) 20 7378 5496
Hepatitis C Advice Line: 0870 242 2467
Web: www.mainliners.org.uk
Newsletter produced bi-monthly for healthcare professionals, service users and anyone who has an interest in drug use, commercial sex work, HIV prevention and hepatitis. Helpline advice and information service for people affected by drug use, HIV and hepatitis.

Medical Council on Alcoholism

3 St. Andrew's Place, Regent's Park, London NW1 4LB.
Telephone: +44(0)20 7487 4445
Email: mca@medicouncilalcol.demon.co.uk
Website: www.medicouncilalcol.demon.co.uk
Charity working to increase knowledge about the effects of alcohol in the medical field.

Methadone Alliance

Room 312 Panther House, 38 Mount Pleasant, London WC1X 0AN.
Helpline: 0207 837 4379 (12 noon and 4pm every weekday, except bank holidays)
Website: www.m-alliance.org.uk
Supports people who receive prescribed drugs for the treatment of their drug dependency.

Narcotics Anonymous
Website: www.ukna.org
Helpline: 0845 3733366
Self-help organisation for people with drug dependencies.

National Addiction Centre
Website: www.iop.kcl.ac.uk/iopweb/departments/home/
default.aspx?locator=346
Established to bring together and network the skills of scientists and
clinicians.

National Association for Premenstrual Syndrome
41 Old Road, East Peckham, Kent TN12 5AP.
Telephone/Fax (UK): 0870 777 2178; (Int): +44(0)1622 872578
Email: contact@pms.org.uk
Website: www.pms.org.uk
UK-based international patient and medical member charity. Advice is
prepared by clinicians and expert patient members to help all those
affected by PMS and menstrual ill-health.

National Centre For Eating Disorders
54 New Road, Esher, Surrey KT10 9NU.
Telephone: 0845 838 2040
Website: www.eating-disorders.org.uk
Provides effective solutions for eating disorders such as compulsive
eating, unsuccessful dieting and bulimia.

National Treatment Agency for Substance Misuse
Website: www.nta.nhs.uk
Special health authority governing substance use treatment in
England. Aims to increase the availability, capacity and effectiveness
of treatment for drug misuse in England. This site includes details of
the NTA's work programme, as well as publications and guidance for
those in the drug treatment sector.

Rehab: What Works
Website: www.eata.org.uk/rehab.php
This is the text of a report from EATA summarising the key research
findings concerning 'what works' in the rehabilitative treatment of
substance dependency.

Release
Website: www.release.org.uk
The national legal and drugs advice and support service. Range of advice and information services in response to people requiring assistance with matters to do with drugs and the law. Primarily aimed at drug users, their families and friends but professionals from a wide range of statutory and voluntary agencies have increasingly used them. Offers a range of specialist services to professionals and the public concerning drugs, the law and human rights.

Re-solv
Website: www.re-solv.org
Helpline: 0808 800 2345
National charity solely dedicated to the prevention of solvent and volatile substance abuse. Information about solvent and volatile substance abuse; factsheets; online training course.

Scottish Drugs Forum
Shaftesbury House, 5 Waterloo Street, Glasgow G2 6AY.
Telephone: 0141 221 1175
Email: enquiries@sdf.org.uk
Website: www.sdf.org.uk
National nongovernmental drugs policy and information agency working in partnership with others to coordinate effective responses to drug use in Scotland. Aims to support and represent, at both local and national levels, a wide range of interests, promoting collaborative, evidence-based responses to drug use.

Society for the Study of Addiction
Executive Office, 19 Springfield Mount, Leeds LS2 9NG.
Telephone: 0113 295 1315
Website: www.addiction-ssa.org
Research organisation in the addiction and addiction treatment field.

Substance Misuse Management in General Practice
Website: www.smmgp.org.uk
Network to support GPs and other members of the primary healthcare team who work with substance misuse in the UK. The project team produces the Substance Misuse Management in General Practice newsletter (Network).

SubstanceMisuse.net
Website: www.substancemisuse.net
This site aims to raise awareness and understanding of substance misuse, the problems it creates and the ways to deal with these problems. It provides: a portal for news on drug and alcohol misuse, from worldwide news media and professional sources; original articles on key issues, personal stories, project profiles, recommended books; content for the general public, practitioners and problem users.

The Advisory Council on Alcohol and Drug Education (TACADE)
6 St Ann's Passage, King Street, Manchester M2 6AD.
Telephone: 0161 836 6850
Email: ho@tacade.co.uk
Website: www.tacade.com
Not-for-profit charitable organisation working in the field of personal, social, health and citizenship education (including drug, alcohol, tobacco and sexual health issues) for children and young people. Increasingly, TACADE works with the more vulnerable, at risk young people.

UK Harm Reduction Alliance
Website: www.ukhra.org
On-line community for people working in harm reduction field.
A campaigning coalition of drug users, health and social care workers, criminal justice workers and educationalists that aims to put public health and human rights at the centre of drug treatment and service provision for drug users.

Index